# MEN'S HEALTH TODAY 2007

# MEN'S HEALTH TODAY 2007

## Everything You Need to Know for Your Best Year Ever

RODALE

© 2007 by Rodale Inc.

Interior photographs: page 1 by Monte Isom; page 31 by Svend Lindback; pages 67–69 by Beth Bischoff; page 79 by Diego Uchitel; page 113 by Augustus Butera; page 145 by Hilmar; page 207 by David Sacks/Getty Images; page 233 by Stefan Nyvang; page 265 by Peter Gerson

ISBN 13: 978-1-59486-534-3
ISBN: 10: 1-59486-534-5

2  4  6  8  10  9  7  5  3  1  hardcover

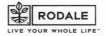

RODALE
LIVE YOUR WHOLE LIFE™

We inspire and enable people to improve their lives and the world around them
For more of our products visit **rodalestore.com** or call 800-848-4735

# CONTENTS

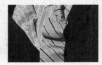

# INTRODUCTION

You're busy, we know, doing 95 in the 55 mph zone of life. But with the scenery whizzing by so fast, there's so much you need to know to be the best that you can be. Unfortunately, you don't have time to stop at a rest area, let alone sit at the computer and research the latest and greatest answers to the questions that come up in your overscheduled life.

So we did the work for you. We talked with experts, read the studies, and tested the products—all so you don't have to. And we crammed into the pages of this book the best advice out there on the topics that matter the most to men: health, fitness, weight loss, fatherhood, work, style, and, of course, sex.

In this book you'll discover how to take advantage of the astonishing new advances in heart care, how to beat the odds against prostate cancer, and how to arm yourself with knowledge about a deadly stroke condition. You'll learn how to burn fat with food, fire up your metabolism, and stay lean for life.

In the section on fatherhood, you'll find out how to decode your teen's secret language, get tips on keeping your kids in shape, and glean some advice from one very famous father. And you'll learn how to unleash your creativity, earn plenty of money for everything, and heed some advice on going into business with a friend in the Work Smarter section.

To help you actually make it in to work each day, take the advice in the Stay Well section. You'll learn easy methods to extinguish heartburn, eliminate ulcers, and solve other digestive dilemmas. You'll also discover six minor health threats that could forewarn of major problems.

You'll be able to do all of these things with more style after reading our Look Great section. Here, we'll keep you from making six common style blunders and share the wisdom of 50 of the nation's top business leaders.

In the Enhance Sex section, you'll find seven triggers that can coax her over the top to ecstasy as well as three simple ways to recharge your sex life. Wondering what the woman in your life is really thinking? We'll take you to the final frontier for an illuminating—and surprising—glimpse inside one woman's brain.

We hope that this book saves you time during your pursuit of your best year ever!

# ONE

# FIGHT FAT

# READ UP ON IT

## The Weight-Loss Rules

With these five simple steps, you'll burn fat with food

**by Phillip Rhodes**

Because most purveyors of weight-loss plans are idiots, the words *diet* and *deprivation* have become nearly synonymous. When you start thinking about reducing your gut, you imagine a dreary patch of flavor denial and an aching belly, and quite naturally you turn away. That's what's wrong with the average diet: It contains the seeds of its own destruction.

We're not going there. Instead, we offer this promise: We'll help you chase your extra 10 or 15 pounds out of town by tempting you with eating opportunities all day long—by keeping your belly so full it'll never occur to you that you're on a diet. And all we ask is that you agree to explore a broader swath of life's big buffet.

The fact is, you can feel better than you do today; you can have more energy; you can improve your long-term health prospects; you can even get lucky more often, with better results. And food—the right kind of food—is your ticket; all the secrets are right here. In 5 weeks, you'll be in your new home: the land of the 32-inch waist. Ready? Let's go.

I mean, let's eat.

### RULE #1: EAT FIVE MEALS A DAY

That's three squares and two snacks. In a study in the *American Journal of Epidemiology*, researchers found that men who ate four or more times a

## TRACK YOUR LOSSES

Research shows that for every pound of weight you lose, you'll melt $\frac{1}{4}$ inch off your waist. Wrap a measuring tape around your abdomen. (For accuracy, the bottom of the tape should touch the tops of your hip bones; your navel will move as you lose weight.) Don't compress the skin.

day had half the risk of becoming overweight compared with those who ate three times or fewer. This doesn't mean three feasts and two 900-calorie "snacks"; read on for the foods to pile on your plate.

## RULE #2: FILL UP ON FIBER

"Fiber is the best food you can eat when you're trying to lose weight," says Gay Riley, RD, a nutritionist in Dallas and author of *Pocket Personal Trainer*. Here's why: It slows your rate of digestion, which keeps you feeling full longer and reduces sugar cravings. And because it binds to other foods, fiber helps hustle calories out of the body. A USDA study determined that people who consume 24 grams of fiber daily earn a 90-calorie free pass. Your goal is 5 grams of fiber at each meal.

Here are some foods with 5 or more grams of fiber:

- 1 cup of any cereal with *bran* in the name—such as raisin bran or All-Bran (If the magic word is missing, check the Nutrition Facts label.)
- 1 cup of cooked beans—pinto, kidney, navy, any kind

Here are some foods with 2 to 4 grams of fiber:

- 1 medium apple, pear, orange, or banana
- 1 cup of any fruit that ends in *berry*
- $\frac{1}{2}$ cup of cooked asparagus, broccoli, brussels sprouts, carrots, cauliflower, green beans, sauerkraut, or spinach
- 1 ounce (about a handful) of almonds, peanuts, cashews, pecans, or sunflower seeds
- 1 cup of cooked brown rice or whole-wheat pasta or two slices of whole-wheat bread

## START TODAY

**Step 1: Clean out your fridge.** And your cabinets. Toss out (or give away) any nondiet soda, any pasta or bread that isn't 100 percent whole wheat, and any cereal that has a cartoon mascot.

**Step 2: Fill it up again.** Build your shopping list using "125 Best Foods" from www.menshealth.com/bestfoods. You'll find dozens of convenient, healthy foods.

**Step 3: Plan meals for 1 week.** By knowing what you're going to eat and when, you'll be more likely to stay on course. Make this a weekly ritual, like watching *Laguna Beach*.

# 3 EASY MEALS YOU CAN MAKE NOW

**Egg Muffins:** Coat a muffin tin with cooking spray and crack 1 egg into each cup. Drop in 1 tablespoon each of diced vegetables and diced deli turkey. Stir. Top with grated cheese. Bake at 350°F for 12 to 15 minutes, let cool, then freeze in zipper-lock bags. To reheat, nuke for 30 seconds.

**Turkey Roll-Ups:** Spread 2 tablespoons of light cream cheese on a 10-inch whole-wheat tortilla. Drop on 2 tablespoons each of diced green onion and chunky salsa. Layer on 4 to 6 slices of deli turkey. Roll. Wrap in plastic wrap and store in the fridge.

**Broccoli and Rice Casserole:** Prepare 1 pouch of quick-cooking brown rice in 2 cups of low-sodium chicken stock. When it's done, stir in 1 cup each of grated low-fat Cheddar cheese and low-fat milk, then 2 cups each of steamed broccoli and chopped smoked pork loin. Add salt and pepper. Cool. Divide into 4 microwave-safe dishes. Freeze. To reheat, zap for 1 minute.

## RULE #3: PUT A LIMIT ON STARCH

Since 1980, the average guy's food intake has grown by 500 calories a day, nearly 80 percent of which can be attributed to carbohydrates; in that time, the prevalence of obesity has increased by 80 percent. The lesson: Cap your intake of the most carbohydrate-dense foods—such as grains and potatoes—at three servings a day. (One serving is the equivalent of one slice of bread, one-half cup of cooked pasta or rice, or one small potato.) Always eat the highest-fiber, least-processed versions of these foods—whole-wheat breads, pastas, and cereals; brown rice instead of white; and whole potatoes, including the skin.

## RULE #4: DON'T COUNT CALORIES

A good diet is effortless. By frequently eating the right foods, you'll eliminate hunger and control your calorie intake.

**Never restrict your produce intake.** You can't eat too many fruits and vegetables, potatoes excepted. Fruits and vegetables contain very few calories, little starch, and lots of fiber.

**Have some protein with every meal.** Make an effort to eat a serving or two of high-quality protein—yogurt, cheese, milk, beef, turkey, chicken, fish, pork, eggs, or nuts. You'll get the daily ideal of 8 grams of leucine, an amino acid that's critical for boosting metabolism and preserving muscle as you drop pounds.

## SIMPLE SWITCHES

**A salty, crunchy fix:** Reach for a pickle, not the Pringles. Dill spears (1 calorie each) will cover both cravings.

**Restaurant sides:** Substitute vegetables for potatoes, pasta, or rice. This drastically reduces calories and keeps insulin levels low.

**At Starbucks:** Opt for fat-free instead of whole milk and avoid beverages with "mocha," "toffee," or "chai" in their names. On average, you'll cut the calorie content by 75 percent.

**Don't be afraid of fat.** Researchers at the City of Hope Medical Center in Duarte, California, report that men who ate a low-calorie, high-fat diet lost 63 percent more weight in 6 months than those who followed a low-fat plan with the same number of calories. By replacing some of the starches with fat—which takes longer to digest—you'll stay full longer and eat less. Emphasize healthy, unsaturated fats: In the study, the high-fat dieters ate 3 ounces of almonds a day.

### RULE #5: RISE AND DINE

Never mind what you've seen at Denny's—fat guys skip breakfast. University of Massachusetts researchers found that men who skip breakfast are 4½ times more likely to be obese than those who don't. "Eating breakfast is like putting kindling on the fire of your metabolism," says Riley, so your body will be less likely to store fat. Make sure you eat within 90 minutes of waking. Men in the study who waited longer increased their chances of obesity by nearly 50 percent.

# The Clock Diet

Eat by the clock to fire up your metabolism and stay lean for life

**by John Berardi, PhD**

The last time it happened, it was the girl who cuts my hair. "So, what kind of diet are you on?" she asked. Since I'm a nutritional biochemist, it's a question I'm used to. My instinct was to skip the scientific details, spit out a four-word answer, and hope she'd move on to the neck shaving. The problem: My diet doesn't fit any of the usual descriptions. It's not low-carb, low-fat, or high-protein. I'm not a vegetarian, and I haven't sworn off sugar. The truth is, I eat almost everything. And that's what makes it so effective.

There are plenty of experts who claim that all that matters is the number of calories you eat: If you want to lose weight, eat fewer calories than you burn. This may make sense on paper, but your body is far more complex than that. You see, it's not just how much you eat; it's what you eat—and when you eat it.

Case in point: carbohydrates. The fast-digesting kind—breads, pasta, rice, potatoes, baked goods, and candy—raise blood sugar quickly. This signals your body to stop burning (and start storing) fat and forces it to use the excess sugar for energy instead. In contrast, slow-digesting carbohydrates, such as fruits and vegetables, keep blood-sugar levels normal, which allows your body to continue to burn fat. So, even though a high-sugar cookie and a big bowl of fruit may have the same number of calories, they have very different effects on your ability to lose body fat.

## TIMING IS EVERYTHING

### Your hour-by-hour eating plan

To burn more fat, add fish oil to any meal. In a study, 3 grams a day boosted metabolism by up to 400 calories. That's enough to lose nearly a pound a week. Our choice: Coromega (www.coromega.com).

**6:30 a.m. breakfast:** Denver omelet (turkey ham, green peppers, and onions, cooked in olive oil) and green tea

**9:30 a.m. snack:** Apple with cheese slices, or a Super Shake (see page 9)

**12:30 p.m. lunch:** Chicken-and-vegetable stir-fry and diet soda

**3:30 p.m. snack:** Cottage cheese or plain yogurt with diced pineapple, or a Super Shake (see page 9)

**6:15 p.m. postworkout drink:** (following 5:30 p.m. workout) 1½ cups chocolate milk

**8:15 p.m. dinner:** Turkey sausage with whole-wheat pasta and spinach salad

But here's what's surprising: High-sugar carbohydrates aren't always bad. In fact, sometimes they're the smartest foods you can eat. The secret is timing. Here's when (and what) you should be eating to build a lean, muscular body—around the clock.

## TIME ZONE 1: RIGHT AFTER YOU WAKE

In a study of 2,831 people, researchers at Harvard University found that people who ate breakfast every day were 44 percent less likely to be overweight and 41 percent less likely to suffer from insulin resistance—a precursor to diabetes—than those who had no morning meal.

**How to eat:** Fill your plate with high-quality protein, slow-digesting carbohydrates, and healthy fats. (See the table below.) The protein stops muscle breakdown and provides the raw materials for laying down new muscle; the carbohydrates replenish energy stores without elevating blood sugar; and healthy fats assure your body that there's more coming in, giving it the green light to burn stored fat.

| High-Quality Protein | Slow-Digesting Carbohydrates | Healthy Fats |
| --- | --- | --- |
| Eggs and egg whites | Oats | Olive oil |
| Lean beef | Onions | Canola oil |
| Turkey | Tomatoes | Fish oil |
| Chicken | Beans | Flaxseeds |
| Fish | Green vegetables | Nuts |
| Low-fat milk | Berries | Sunflower seeds |
| Low-fat cheese | Oranges | Olives |
| Plain, low-fat yogurt | Apples | Avocados |

## TIME ZONE 2: EVERY 3 HOURS AFTER BREAKFAST

Waiting more than 4 or 5 hours between meals causes your blood sugar to bottom out, leaving you weak, irritable, and tired. (For the record, both high and low blood sugar can be problematic.) To combat this, your body secretes cortisol, a hormone that boosts blood-sugar levels back to normal.

YEAR WHEN EVERY AMERICAN WILL BE OBESE IF OBESITY RATES CONTINUE TO RISE AS THEY HAVE OVER THE PAST 25 YEARS: 2058

# THE SUPER SHAKE

### Your recipe for the healthiest meal replacement on the planet

The metabolism-boosting power of this liquid snack is unrivaled: Substitute it for 2 cups of microwave buttered popcorn and 16 ounces of soda just once a day, and you'll lose weight—without making any other changes to your diet. The bonus: A Super Shake provides you with more nutrition in one gulp than most of your co-workers take in all day. Just blend all the ingredients together for 60 seconds, pour, and drink. (Don't worry; it tastes good.)

**1 cup green tea:** This no-calorie beverage has been shown to boost metabolism.

**1 scoop casein protein:** Because casein is a slow-digesting type of milk protein, it'll provide a steady supply of protein to your muscles for hours. We like Metabolic Drive Super Protein Shake (www.t-nation.com).

**1 tablespoon ground flaxseed:** Flaxseed is a healthy fat that's been shown to lower LDL cholesterol, triglycerides, and blood pressure in lab animals. Buy it preground at a health food store.

**1/2 cup frozen raspberries, blackberries, or strawberries:** Packed with disease-fighting antioxidants, these fiber-filled fruits are three of the best foods known.

**1 tablespoon mixed nuts:** Research shows that adding one or two handfuls of nuts to your daily diet reduces your risk of heart disease without leading to weight gain.

**1 tablespoon Greens+:** The nutrient equivalent of six servings of fruits and vegetables a day, it's the best-kept secret in supplements (www.greensplus.com).

Trouble is, one of the ways it does this is by converting muscle protein to sugar, what exercise scientists call *muscle wasting*, two words you never want to see paired. The solution: frequent meals. Eating more often helps regulate blood-sugar levels, protecting your muscles from being broken down and used as energy. Here's a bonus: South African researchers found that men who ate the most frequently consumed 27 percent fewer calories than those who ate the least often.

**How to eat:** As with breakfast, always include protein, along with either healthy fats or slow-digesting carbohydrates (preferably both). Protein is the major player here, since up to 30 percent of its calories are burned during digestion, compared with 8 percent of carbohydrates and 2 percent of fats. Keep in mind that the recommendations for this time zone may include

**PERCENTAGE GREATER SEXUAL DESIRE FELT
BY THIN MEN THAN BY FAT ONES: 240**

snacks, lunch, and even dinner, depending on the time of day you exercise. For a fail-safe snack or meal, check out "The Super Shake" on the previous page.

## TIME ZONE 3: AFTER YOUR WORKOUT

Unlike before your workout, fast-digesting carbs are now more desirable than the slow-digesting type. That's because an intense workout changes your body's priorities: As sugar is absorbed into your bloodstream, it's preferentially shuttled to your muscles—instead of being used as fuel—and is stored there for later use. The kicker is that this forces your body to accelerate the rate at which it burns fat for energy.

**How to eat:** Combine high-quality protein with fast-digesting carbohydrates at two separate times.

First, immediately after you finish exercising: Ideally, this should be a liquid meal, to speed the absorption of protein and carbohydrates into your bloodstream. Researchers at the University of Texas Medical Branch found that 6 grams of essential amino acids and 35 grams of carbohydrates are an ideal combination for promoting muscle growth after exercise. That's almost identical to 12 ounces of chocolate milk.

Second, 2 hours later: This time, opt for solid food. That is, consider this the best time to eat spaghetti and meatballs—guilt-free. Even better, combine fast- and slow-digesting carbs with protein by choosing a lean meat and a green vegetable to go along with pasta, rice, or a potato. Once you've eaten this meal, follow the guidelines in Time Zone 2 for the rest of the day.

**One caveat:** If you exercise first thing in the morning (before breakfast), have your postworkout drink prior to working out, follow the guidelines for eating 2 hours after exercise, and then resume the recommendations for the rest of the day (Time Zone 2).

# Saboteur-Busting Secrets

Exercise your willpower with this temptation-proof plan

**by Allison Winn Scotch**

Nobody's the innocent victim of a drive-thru feeding. But you're not entirely to blame for the extra pie in your gut, either. Your shape-up strategy may be secretly under attack—from your friends, your family, and even the chemicals in your brain. Identify the saboteurs behind your diet's demise, and then learn how to sabotage them.

## THE SABOTEUR: YOUR STRESS

In stressful situations, levels of the hormone cortisol spike, and that tells your body to go into fat-storing mode. Eat fatty food and watch the damage multiply.

**Fix your head.** Identify the type of stress you're under, says Jim Karas, author of *The Business Plan for the Body*. "Is it temporary, like a bar exam, or more permanent, like your job?" Short-term stress will pass. Long-term stress may require a more permanent solution, such as a new job.

**Fix your routine.** Make healthy eating effortless. If you don't buy pints of ice cream, they won't be lurking in your freezer, sending siren calls in the middle of the night. Eat one serving of protein-rich almonds (about 24), which can help level off the highs and lows associated with stress. Or pick up a container of plain oats; a half-cup serving contains 4 grams of fiber along with some melatonin, a calming hormone that's related to sleep. Plan B: Take a short, but fast, run around the block or hit an afternoon kickboxing class. High-intensity workouts help relieve tension, but they also provide a much greater calorie afterburn than low-intensity exercise like walking or slow jogging, Karas says.

**NUMBER OF TIMES MORE LIKELY WEIGHT-LOSS SURGERY IS TO RESULT IN DEATH FOR A MAN THAN A WOMAN: 3**

## THE SABOTEUR: YOUR WIFE

Though it's tempting, don't blame your beloved for your belly. This would be (a) wrong and (b) reasonable defense at her trial. But know this: Researchers at the University of Minnesota found that men and women usually gain 6 to 8 pounds in the first 2 years of marriage. "Once you're married, that need to impress is gone," says Edward Abramson, PhD, author of *Marriage Made Me Fat!* "You may go to the gym less often, go out for meals or to parties more frequently, and develop new rituals, such as sitting on the couch together snacking."

**Fix your head.** Regain a little bit of that need to impress. What would your single self say—the one whose good looks and moxie helped convince her to marry you? As for that shared bowl of extra-butter popcorn, Dr. Abramson says, ask yourself, "Why am I eating?" Boredom? Habit? Better yet, don't even bring those binge foods into the house.

**Fix your routine.** Get off the couch, get out of your rut, and lose the remote. Instead of watching *Access Hollywood* after dinner, keep your mind occupied and your hands busy: Read a book, surf the Web, or organize a fam-

# THE ULTIMATE WEIGHT-LOSS WEAPON

Atkins is tired and The Zone is out of bounds. Embrace your bran flakes, because roughage will soon be all the rage. Fiber is the next big diet craze.

Need proof? Food manufacturing giant ConAgra recently developed a fiber-filled whole-wheat flour that's fine-grained enough to replace white flour in pastries and other baked goods. Products using the stuff—called Ultragrain—will be in stores soon. So will two varieties of FiberChoice sweets: orange-flavored candies that deliver 2 grams of fiber, and chewable wafers in apple, grape, and strawberry flavors that pack 4 grams.

Beth Kunkel, PhD, a professor of food science at Clemson University, explains that fiber blocks calorie absorption by keeping the intestines from breaking down the caloric parts of your food.

To get your roughage requirement (20 to 35 grams per day), check food labels for the word *whole*, as in *whole wheat* or *whole grain* (average of 3 grams of fiber per $1/2$ cup); eat the skin on your veggies (2 to 3 grams per $1/2$ cup); get your fruit from fresh or frozen (2 grams per piece or $1/2$ cup) but not juice, which is virtually fiber-free; and eat a bowl of fiber-rich cereal. Easy fiber sources include black beans (15 grams per cup), "health-food" cereals like Fiber One (14 grams per $1/2$ cup), whole-wheat pasta (4 grams per cup), green beans (3.5 grams per cup), brown rice (4 grams per cup), or a medium apple (4 grams). Not to mention Grandma's Metamucil. "Fiber is fiber," Dr. Kunkel says.

ily card game. Or, surprise her with a round of everyone's favorite indoor sport (which burns an average of about 2 calories per minute—you do the math). Check out www.caloriesperhour.com for a wide variety of activities and their associated caloric burn. And when you're ready to cool down, try an Italian water ice (120 calories per cup) instead of ice cream (290 calories per cup).

## THE SABOTEUR: YOUR KIDS

Having adorable offspring in the house sharply increases the likelihood of Combos in the cupboard—some of which inevitably end up in your mouth. In putting their kids first, dads tend to skip breakfast, grab unhealthy snacks, and overlook exercise.

**Fix your head.** See the future. That sugary snack that your kids burn off in an hour will haunt you as a fat deposit.

**Fix your routine.** Plan every day's meals—including snacks—so that you're always eating healthy foods, such as berries, yogurt, whole-wheat toast with peanut butter, and nuts. "A healthy diet never happens by accident," says Melinda Johnson, RD, spokeswoman for the American Dietetic Association. You can still make junk food a once-a-week thing. Designate Friday as Fruity Pebbles day, for example.

## THE SABOTEUR: LATE-NIGHT TV

Not getting enough deep sleep inhibits production of growth hormones, which could lead to premature symptoms of middle age, such as abdominal obesity, reduced muscle mass and strength, and diminished exercise capacity. In short: You become your grandfather overnight.

**Fix your head.** Don't plot a staffing reorganization before bed. Establish a ritual that signals your body that the day is over 30 minutes before you're ready to hit the sack. Turn off the computer, read, stretch, or set the TV volume low, Karas says.

**Fix your routine.** Exercise in the morning or afternoon, says Eric Nofzinger, MD, an expert in sleep disorders at the University of Pittsburgh School of Medicine. Evening workouts may leave you too stimulated to sleep, so instead, develop a clear end-of-day habit. Snuggle with your wife while she's watching *Desperate Housewives*. Let Susan and company put you to sleep—in seconds. Trust us.

## THE SABOTEUR: YOUR PRESCRIPTIONS

Prozac may cure your mental woes, but it can also doom your diet. "Antidepressants affect weight by regulating serotonin, which is involved in both mood and appetite," says Scott Isaacs, PhD, of the Emory School of Medicine in Atlanta and author of *Hormonal Balance*. Top culprits include Zoloft, Paxil, and nonmood-altering drugs such as Benadryl and most diabetes medications.

**Fix your head.** Consider having it shrunk. "Too many people take antidepressant medications instead of addressing the issues in their lives that are contributing to the depression," Dr. Isaacs says. Talking to a mental-health professional may prove more effective than pill popping, and there are definitely no side effects.

**Fix your routine.** Ask your doctor about switching your medications. Alternative meds may better suit your chemical makeup without the puffy side effects. "Also, by being aware of the increases in appetite associated with antidepressant medications, you can eat lower-calorie foods to satisfy your appetite and not gain weight," Dr. Isaacs says. Try fat-free popcorn in the afternoon or foods high in fiber (fruits and vegetables) or protein (nuts and milk) to help keep you full.

## THE SABOTEUR: YOUR FRIENDS

Pals can make or break a weight-loss plan. Sometimes it's innocent enough—maybe your best friend suggests ditching the gym for a boys' night out. Or maybe a not-so-good friend deliberately tries to sabotage your diet: "Oh come on, let's order the cheese fries with this pitcher." An occasional stumble won't cause any harm, but giving in all the time will.

**Fix your head.** Ask for help. "Let people know how to help you, and many will," says Beth Kitchin, assistant professor of nutritional sciences at the University of Alabama at Birmingham. Friends who unwittingly lead you into temptation will stop. And you'll undermine the efforts of those false friends, too.

**Fix your routine.** Eat a bowl of Frosted Mini-Wheats with low-fat milk before you go out. The fiber will keep you feeling full, the sugar will satisfy your craving for mudslides, and the calcium will help you burn fat even while you're sitting at the bar.

# S C I - G U Y

## Aim High

Most experts recommend setting modest weight-reduction goals, but a new study from the University of Minnesota suggests that having high weight-loss expectations may help you lose a greater amount of weight. The researchers found that men who tried to lose an average of 16 percent of their body weight—instead of the commonly recommended 5 to 10 percent—did indeed drop more than their conservative counterparts. "They seem to understand that it takes more effort to lose more weight," speculates Jennifer Linde, PhD, the lead researcher. Make your overall goal as lofty as you like—20, 30, or even 50 pounds—but set a practical time frame, capping expectations at an average loss of 1 pound a week.

## Pack on Protein

When McMaster University scientists assessed the food intake of 617 people, they found that eating more protein may reduce the fat around your midsection. People who ate 20 grams more protein every day than the group average had 6 percent lower waist-to-hip ratios. Most made small adjustments, such as replacing ¾ cup of rice with half a chicken breast, says Anwar Merchant, PhD, lead researcher.

## Spice It Up

Start your meal with something spicy. Researchers in the Netherlands found that eating hot peppers may help you eat less. In the study, 12 men ate 0.9 gram of ground chile peppers—in pill form or mixed into a tomato-juice

**NUMBER OF TIMES AN OBESE PERSON THAN A THIN PERSON IS MORE LIKELY TO DIE AFTER EXPERIENCING A CRITICAL INJURY: 6**

beverage—30 minutes before getting a free run at an all-you-can-eat buffet. Compared with a placebo, the pill helped men cut their food intake by 10 percent, while the liquid mixture resulted in a 16 percent reduction. The pepper-primed eaters chose less calorie-dense foods, says study author Margriet Westerterp, PhD. Get your meal off to a searing start with an extra-spicy Bloody Mary or a cup of chili spiked with Tabasco.

## Order the Soup

Turns out chicken soup isn't just good for your soul; it's good for your abs. Researchers at Pennsylvania State University found that snacking on soup can help speed weight loss. The study tracked 147 men and women who followed reduced-calorie diets for a year; those who ate one serving of soup twice a day lost 50 percent more weight than those who ate healthful but carbohydrate-heavy snacks, such as baked chips or crackers. Creamy clam chowder doesn't count, says lead researcher Barbara Rolls, PhD. You want broth-based soups. Try the chicken-noodle or vegetable-beef varieties of Campbell's microwavable Soup at Hand; each contains less than 100 calories.

## Have a Cuppa

Sure, diet soda is calorie-free carbonation. But if you want a beverage that can actually burn blubber instead of blocking it, drink brewed green tea instead. In fact, green tea may be a more effective fat fighter than previously thought. The credit goes to catechins, chemicals found in varying levels in green tea. In a recent Japanese study, men who drank tea high in catechins lost nearly 5 pounds, compared with no drop in weight for men who drank an ordinary brew. Lead researcher Ichiro Tokimitsu, PhD, suggests that the catechins may help hustle fat molecules out of the bloodstream before they're deposited around your middle. Drink three 15-ounce servings of green tea a day to start losing the lard, he says.

## Don't Stop

Serious science and underwear rarely cross paths. So you may have already heard about a recent study from the Mayo Clinic showing that fidgeting burns more calories than previously thought. When researchers equipped 20 people with high-tech drawers that monitored slight levels of movement 120

**PERCENTAGE OF AMERICANS WHO DON'T BELIEVE OBESE PEOPLE ARE TO BLAME FOR THEIR WEIGHT:**

# 64

times a minute, 24 hours a day, for 10 days, they found that overweight people simply moved less than their lean counterparts, burning 350 fewer calories per day. What you may not have heard, though, is how to make the calorie-burning power of fidgeting work for you: Trade your office chair for a Swiss ball. "Use it instead of a desk chair for 15 to 20 minutes every hour," says sports-performance coach Charles Staley, CSCS. Not only will the ball keep you in perpetual motion, but it'll also strengthen your core muscles, alleviating another side effect of too much sitting: back pain.

## Blame Your Poor Taste

Can't seem to shed the flab? The reason may be on the tip of your tongue. A new Rutgers University study shows that your taste buds could hold the secret to controlling your weight. Researchers discovered that people with a dulled sense of taste have body-mass indexes (BMIs) 2.5 points higher than those who experience flavors fully. Part of the explanation, says Beverly Tepper, PhD, lead researcher, is that folks with less-sensitive taste buds prefer foods that are intensely sweet or fatty, which often are also high in calories. How can you tell what kind of taster you are? If eating jalapeño chile peppers makes you break out in a sweat, then your tongue is plenty sensitive. If you barely notice peppers' heat, then you're the person artificial sweeteners were made for. Pick up faux-sugar versions of sweet foods or try substituting salty baked pretzels for your favorite chips.

## Raid Right

Conan O'Brien viewers, take note: You may no longer have to feel guilty about late-night snacking, say Danish scientists. In a 6-year study of more than 2,100 people, the researchers found that weight changes in men who regularly woke up and raided the fridge were similar to those in men who did not eat during the night, regardless of what the snackers scarfed down. (Some female snackers gained as much as 10 pounds.) Lead researcher Berit Heit-mann, PhD, suggests that men may be better than women at regulating their calorie intake throughout the day, and so might be less likely to binge when they satisfy a craving. That said, try to eat a bowl of oatmeal instead of left-over pizza: The fiber in the oats will fill you up, and their supply of the sleep hormone melatonin will help you conk back out.

## Drink Up

We're all familiar with the weighty consequences of drinking too much beer. Extra calories from alcohol can add up to a Bridgestone-shaped belly. But there is a foam-flecked silver lining. New research shows that moderate beer and wine consumption may help fight diabetes, high blood pressure, and other diseases brought on by excess weight. In a recent study at Boston Med-ical Center, people who consumed 20 such drinks a month were 66 percent less likely to be diagnosed with an obesity-related condition than those who abstained. Study author Matthew Freiberg, MD, speculates that alcohol's ability to raise HDL (good) cholesterol and lower insulin resistance may be responsible. Not all types of alcohol had the same effect, he adds; beer appeared to provide more of a benefit than hard liquor.

## Hold Your Nose

Would-be dieters might want to stay out of sniffing distance of their favorite restaurants. Scent triggers a powerful physiological response that can sabo-tage your diet, according to new research into ghrelin, a hormone that sends "feed me" signals from your stomach to your brain. In an Italian study of 16 people, researchers found that those who saw, smelled, and briefly tasted food experienced the same surge in ghrelin as those who actually chowed down. "There is an anticipatory response to stimulation by palatable foods," reports study author Maura Arosio, PhD. In other words, you're as Pavlovian as a pooch. That's fine when you're planning to eat anyway. But if you're an impulse eater, try to stay upwind of potentially triggering aromas.

# WHAT'S NEW

## Not-So-Fun House Mirror

Imagine a mirror that shows what you may look like in 5 years' time. French scientists are developing one that uses cameras placed around your home to record your activities (or lack thereof). The information is sent to a computer, which calculates the cumulative effect of your behavior on your body and then displays the result on the screen. Prototypes could be available this year.

## The Next Magic Weight-Loss Pill

A prescription antismoking drug called Acomplia (rimonabant) shows promise. It blocks the brain's cannabinoid receptors. Cannabis smokers and obese people both experience extreme hunger, so it's thought that blocking these receptors suppresses appetite. The drug was approved for use in Europe in February 2006, but the FDA declined final approval for use in the United States until a number of unspecified issues were resolved.

## Outpatient Gastric Bypass Surgery

Gastric bypass is increasingly done as a minimally invasive laparoscopic operation and may soon become an outpatient procedure, says *Men's Health* weight-loss advisor David Katz, MD. We'll probably see it combined with drug or hormone therapy in the near future, he predicts. But it's better to prevent obesity in the first place—going under the knife is a last resort.

## Calorie-Burning Beverages

No-calorie drinks are now the diet norm, but new product developments may soon yield negative-calorie beverages. At a recent medical conference, Elite FX, a Florida-based company, presented its study demonstrating that its caffeinated Celsius diet beverage raised participants' metabolic rates by nearly 15 percent—three times the boost from another popular diet drink. Researchers say the effect probably was produced by the known metabolism boosters caffeine and green tea. Celsius is now sold in Alabama, Florida, and Louisiana and online at www.drinkcelsius.com.

## Body Composition Monitor

Body fat is a poor conductor, as Kirstie Alley happily learned when she Godzilla'd the electric fence around her bonbon stash. An impedance scale employs that principle to measure body fat: A low-level current assesses bone density, muscle mass, and the visceral fat padding your midsection. Check out the Tanita BC-533 Innerscan Body-Composition Monitor. This scale even politely suggests a daily calorie intake. For accuracy, it can't match calipers or a dunk tank, but it's consistent enough for weekly progress checks. (Checking more frequently is kind of obsessive.)

# T A K E 5

## Lose Your Gut

Five ways to build your abs fast

What if your boss told you to gain 20 pounds of muscle and lose a third of your body fat? Most of us would end up in the unemployment line, but Ryan Reynolds did as he was told to prepare for his role as a cute vampire killer in *Blade: Trinity*. Here are his tips for sculpting a six-pack—on a full stomach.

**Eat more.** "I attribute my results mostly to nutrition," Reynolds says. He ate every 2 to 3 hours to burn more fat. "Your body doesn't need to store fat for energy if you're feeding it all the time," explains Bobby Strom, Reynolds's LA-based trainer.

**Mix it up.** "I gained a lot more muscle mass when I went on creatine," says Reynolds. He also took L-glutamine, conjugated linoleic acid (CLA), whey, and a multivitamin.

**Go for bulk.** Reynolds doesn't have a personal chef, so he cooks meals in advance. For instance, he'll make a large supply of Irish steel-cut oatmeal and freeze it. That way, the most important meal of the day requires the least work.

**Carve with carbs.** "Never do any of that carve-starve crap," Reynolds says. Instead, watch the clock. He ate most of his carbohydrates postworkout, and none after 8:00 p.m.

**Think about yourself.** "If you hate your workout, you're not going to do it," explains Reynolds. Customize your fitness plan to meet your needs. He found it "meditative" to do ab exercises first instead of last.

# MEN'S HEALTH QUIZ

## Are You Destined for a Six-Pack or a Thirty-Six-Pack?

Take this test to avoid a soft underbelly

**1. Your stress level is...**
A. Redlining
B. Medium hot
C. Jimmy Buffetesque

Loosen up to tighten your belt. Whether you're stressing over your job, your family, or the Clippers' turnover ratio, you're spouting extra cortisol—a hormone that regulates fat metabolism. More cortisol equals more fat, according to Louis Aronne, MD, director of the Comprehensive Weight Control Program in New York City. Worse yet, research from the University of California at San Francisco shows that your abdomen is cortisol-bloat central. Because there's so much blood pumping there, it's four times more likely than the rest of your body to store stress-induced fat. A recent Canadian study found that men who lifted weights had significantly lower levels of cortisol than endurance athletes did. Lifting will help you lose weight, too. Research from Johns Hopkins shows that resistance training makes you burn calories for close to 2 hours after a workout. Jogging increases metabolism for less than an hour. If you hate iron more than infomercials, run hills. It's like weight lifting your body mass.

**2. Tuesday and Thursday are your abs days. How do you work them?**
A. Crunches with a twist
B. Old-fashioned situps
C. That ab-training thingy I bought on the Internet

Bolster your fitness. The bicycle maneuver (pumping your legs while rotating your torso) is the most efficient way to sculpt your midsection, according to a study sponsored by the American Council on Exercise. The next-best exercises are Swiss-ball crunches and exercises using a captain's chair (a gym apparatus that braces your arms so you can raise your knees). If you want to work more muscles, follow the advice from researchers at the Medical College of Georgia, who determined which ab exercises are the most strenuous for the whole body. The answer: full situps from the floor, which activate muscles in the abdomen, back, shoulders, hips, and legs. Second place: basic floor crunches, and third: situps on a Swiss ball. As for those ab-training gadgets—maybe it's time you began exercising your common sense. You can't buy abs with a credit card. It takes work.

### 3. Your love life is...
A. A high-stakes game of chase and be chased
B. A steady commitment I'm settling into
C. Till death do us part (Don't say the words *ball and chain*.)

Spice up your workout and your sex life. The average 180-pound man will gain 6 to 8 pounds in the first 2 years of marriage, according to University of Minnesota researchers. Why? He doesn't need to impress the steady squeeze. (Now hear this: A recent poll showed that 44 percent of women feel that a partner's excess pounds "detrimentally affect the relationship.") Dr. Aronne advises using a partnership to chase the chub: "Instead of plopping down on the couch together, be each other's motivator to get outside and exercise." If your ability levels don't match, don't worry. You can hit the weights at the gym while she takes that goofy Salsarobics class, or she can ride a bike and pass the water bottle while you do your half-marathon prep. The most important thing: Set your date for exercise, then stick to it. Likewise, if the two of you always eat together, you can learn to eat lean together.

### 4. When she asks, "When will you be home from work?" you answer...
A. "Standard day today, baby—9 to 5."
B. "Keep dinner warm. I should be a little late."
C. "I'm on nights this week. See you in the morning."

Work less, live more. Data from the New York Obesity Research Center shows that people who switch to a night shift gain an average of 9.5 pounds. Late-shift work throws off your circadian rhythms and stresses your body, says Dr. Aronne. People exercise less and wind up eating two suppers—one during their time on the job and another after work, before crashing. They're committing a major diet foul. "Don't eat a huge meal right before bed," says Dr. Aronne. "Have dinner with your family before leaving for work, eat small while there, and take some time to relax when you get home. When you wake up the next day, eat a full breakfast." If you're lucky enough to stay on the day shift, watch those late nights that keep you away from your family: Regular mealtimes control cravings, and studies have shown that families who eat together stay skinny together.

### 5. How often do you hit your local happy hour?
A. Rarely (But when I go, I go hog wild.)
B. A few nights a week, but just for a couple of beers
C. Every night (You can't be too happy.)

Party without consequence. Occasional binge drinkers have more abdominal fat than people who consume the same amount but drink regularly, according to a study from the University of Buffalo. So go ahead and claim your regular seat at the bar, but set a limit: Men who drink more than three or four drinks per bar visit have the highest measures of ab flab. One reason: More booze means less testosterone—your muscle-building, libido-boosting hormone. The standard nonprescription remedy for that: Add iron. But don't swallow it. Lift it over your head, repeatedly. Boosting protein intake (with dairy products, low-fat cuts of meat, and whey powder) can also up the amount of high-test in your veins. As for what to order from the barkeep, note that wine drinkers carry the least abdominal fat, while liquor drinkers have the most. Moderate beer swilling wasn't associated with more abdominal fat. (But 5 daily pints of the amber nectar can stunt sperm growth, and 10 pints a day could stop it completely.)

### 6. How do you sleep at night?
A. Eight hours, like clockwork
B. Sometimes great, sometimes not so great
C. I never get what I need

Rest, relax, recharge. A lack of deep sleep alters the production of growth hormones, which might lead to an early case of old age: abdominal obesity,

**AVERAGE AMOUNT OF NET WORTH INCREASE IN OVERWEIGHT MEN WHO SLIMMED DOWN:**

# $4,085

reduced muscle mass and strength, and diminished exercise capability, according to a study from the University of Chicago. "Growth-hormone levels are closely related to fitness levels," says Orfeu Buxton, PhD, of the Harvard Medical School's Division of Sleep Medicine. "Improving fitness also improves sleep and could lead to some weight loss. That would reduce the severity of overweight-related sleep disorders, like sleep apnea." To protect your exercise-induced snooze, don't work out right before bedtime. Allow a few hours for your heart rate to slow.

### Scoring Your Core

| | | | |
|---|---|---|---|
| 1. | A = 3 | B = 2 | C = 1 |
| 2. | A = 1 | B = 2 | C = 3 |
| 3. | A = 3 | B = 2 | C = 1 |
| 4. | A = 1 | B = 2 | C = 3 |
| 5. | A = 3 | B = 1 | C = 2 |
| 6. | A = 1 | B = 3 | C = 2 |

**6 to 9 points**—You're well centered.
**10 to 14 points**—Your six-pack is in sight, if not in hand.
**15 to 18 points**—You're off center.

# BURNING QUESTIONS

**You always say a man's body fat needs to be below 10 percent to see his abs. But what is a good body-fat percentage for general health?**

Healthy body composition can vary from 10 to as high as 25 percent fat, says Tim Lohman, PhD, professor of physiology at the University of Arizona. With greater than 25 percent fat, health risks climb. "If your body fat is over 25 percent, aim to lose 10 percent of your weight and maintain it long-term," he says. A word of advice to manorexics: There's such a thing as too little body fat. Less than 5 percent can jeopardize your immune system.

**I always want to scarf the whole basket of bread at restaurants. Am I addicted to carbs?**

You're just hungry. Curb the impulse by snacking 2 hours before going out. Then order a salad or shrimp cocktail as soon as you sit down.

If you must try the bread, take one slice and pass the basket to the other side of the table or have it taken away. If someone objects, he wins; the basket stays right by his plate.

**Is an unhealthy breakfast better than no breakfast at all?**

Yes—not that you have free rein to order the Meat Lover's Skillet every morning. But there's a whole lot of gray area between a fruit-laden bowl of oatmeal and several pounds of grease and meat, and most of it is preferable to starting the day on an empty stomach. "A latte would probably be better than nothing, because at least you're getting vitamin D and calcium from the milk," says Mark Pereira, PhD, an epidemiologist at the University of Minnesota who studies breakfast habits. Even foods with no redeeming nutritional value, like doughnuts, curb your appetite for a little while. "Skipping breakfast altogether may make you hungrier and lead you to overeat," says Dr. Pereira, so try to eat something. Just don't use it as an excuse to binge.

**Am I better off eating before or after I do my workout, which includes lifting and aerobic exercise, like running?**

The number one rule for performance nutrition is to eat every 3 hours throughout the day, which means you'll be eating before and after every workout. Since you'll eat five or six times a day, no single meal will likely be large enough to interfere with exercise. So don't sweat your preworkout meal; anything less than 500 calories is fine.

But when it comes to postworkout eating, you need to be more precise. Your best move right after a workout is to drink a shake containing protein and carbohydrates, but little or no fat. An example is Biotest Surge (www. biotestedge.com). This type of shake speeds amino acids and sugars to your depleted muscles, which will greatly enhance the results you'll get from your workout. Here's another tip: 2 to 3 hours after exercise is the best time to enjoy some of those bad carbohydrates you've been craving. During that window of opportunity, your body can't put those sugars into fat storage around your waist.

### What contributes the most calories to Americans' diets?

White bread used to be America's main source of energy, but a study by Tufts University found that soda and other sweetened drinks are now the main culprits. In preliminary research, two-thirds of study respondents admitted to getting more calories from sweet drinks than from anything else. We've been saying it for years, and we'll say it again: Switch to water and watch your waistline shrink.

### What should I look for in a nutrition bar?

Like everything else, it's about finding the right balance.

Energy bars supply and replenish energy stores before, during, or after exercise. Look for a 3-to-1 carb-to-protein ratio. "Research has shown that ratio to enhance performance and endurance," says Amanda Carlson, MS, RD, performance-nutrition manager for Athletes' Performance, in Tempe, Arizona. "It will give you the carbohydrates you need to sustain and replenish energy, and enough protein to help repair your muscles." Best bet: Clif Bar (www.clifbar.com).

Protein bars support muscle growth and recovery following strength training. Look for a 2-to-1 carb-to-protein ratio. Avoid bars that have the ratio reversed, as they won't supply enough carbs to replenish energy stores. And choose one that contains both casein and whey protein. A study at Baylor University found that men who consumed this combination gained 50 percent more muscle than those who consumed whey alone. Best bet: EAS Myoplex Deluxe Nutrition (www.eas.com).

Meal-replacement bars serve as a quick, low-calorie meal for dieters or people on the go. If you're eating three meals a day, you want a bar that supplies roughly a third of your daily nutrients. Look for 10 to 30 grams of protein, 30 to 50 grams of carbs, an array of vitamins and minerals, and at least 300 calories. "You also want 5 or more grams of fiber to slow digestion," says Carlson. "That will help you feel full longer and stabilize your energy levels." Best bet: Chef Jay's Tri-O-Plex (www.chefjays.com).

**I've read that when you're trying to drop body fat, you shouldn't eat later than 6:00 p.m. But when I eat early, I find that I'm starving by 8:30. What can I do?**

Sure, your metabolism slows during the evening hours, so you don't want to pig out late at night. But eating something small before you go to bed can actually help you lose weight. Here's why: If you are training hard, going too long between meals can lead to muscle breakdown. Muscle, remember, revs up your metabolism. So keep your muscle fueled by eating a small snack (250 to 400 calories) containing slow-releasing forms of protein, such as poultry or cottage cheese, just before bedtime. This strategy will accelerate your fat loss. My late-night snack is often a scoop of protein powder mixed into a 6-ounce container of plain yogurt.

**I put salt on my bland weight-loss foods to make them easier to eat. Am I making a mistake?**

Yes. Anyone who's peeled back the foil on a bubbling pile of green mush can sympathize, but try other spices—garlic, ginger, turmeric, pepper, or thyme—instead. Or add lemon or lime, balsamic vinegar, or fresh herbs such as cilantro or basil. Unless you're an active athlete sweating sodium when you exercise, reducing your sodium intake is beneficial. It'll also help prevent the bloating that may occur with too much salt intake.

**Lots of diets say you can eat whatever you want 1 day a week. So can I have a few bad things, or can I totally binge?**

Weight isn't the only issue here. It takes a 3,500-calorie surplus to pack on 1 pound, so you'd have to chow down to notice an effect. The real worry is that even one high-fat, high-carbohydrate load can boost oxidative stress in the body and make it harder to resist new temptations. The bottom line: Cheating on your diet doesn't mean abandoning it entirely. Limit your splurge to a few forbidden snacks.

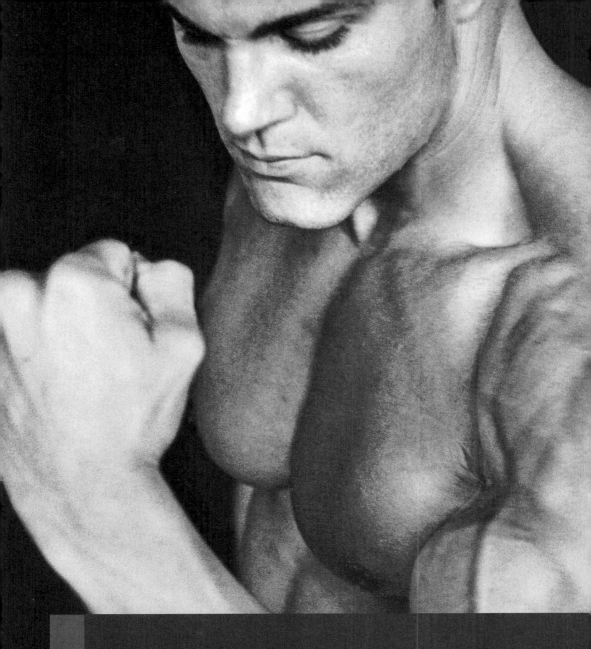

# TWO

# GET FIT

# READ UP ON IT

## The Fountain of Youth

Eight age-proofing reasons why every man should lift weights

**by Adam Campbell**

Indulge us for a moment by flexing your right arm.

Assuming you have an average build—and trust us, you do—your arm is packing about 5 pounds of muscle. It represents nearly 10 percent of the total muscle on your body.

Now, imagine that muscle gone. No biceps, no triceps—only a jiggly mass of skin and fat covering your bones from your shoulder down to your fingertips. That 5 pounds of muscle is about the same amount most men lose between the ages of 24 and 50. And that number doubles by the time they're 60. In fact, once a man passes the half-century mark, he can expect to lose 1 percent of his muscle each year for the rest of his life.

That is, unless he does something about it.

And there's good reason for intervention: The natural erosion of muscle and strength that comes with aging leads directly to weak bones, stiff joints, and a slumped posture and increases your risk of developing heart disease, diabetes, and a host of other maladies. But there's no reason you can't maintain a healthy, strong musculature well into your nineties if you use man's most effective antiaging weapon: resistance training. "Lifting weights regularly signals your body to fight to keep your muscle," says Jeff Volek, PhD, RD, exercise and diet researcher at the University of Connecticut. That means a longer, healthier life. And we can prove it. Here's why every guy should be lifting weights even if he doesn't give a damn about the size of his biceps.

### LIFTING IS GOOD FOR THE GRAY MATTER

Researchers at the University of Michigan found that men who performed three total-body weight workouts per week for 2 months lowered their blood-pressure readings by an average of 8 points. That's enough to reduce the risk of a stroke by 40 percent.

(continued on page 36)

# THE 20-MINUTE TOTAL-BODY WORKOUT

### A time-efficient plan for a longer, healthier, stronger life

Let's get something straight: You're not lifting for the beach or to try to intimidate your daughter's dates. Your goal is efficiency, so you need to focus on exercises that work the most muscle in the least time, says Michael Mejia, CSCS, trainer and author of *Scrawny to Brawny*. As a rule, Mejia recommends only multijoint movements, which force you to bend at more than one joint. Plan your workout around these six basic movements, and you'll train every muscle in your body in less than 20 minutes per session. "It only takes two sets of each movement, done twice a week, to get most of the health benefits of lifting, including maintenance of your muscle and strength," says Mejia. Choose one exercise from each movement category below, and then create your own workout regimen by using the Rules of Repetition on page 39.

## Movement 1

**Quad-dominant:** Any lower-body exercise in which your quadriceps work the hardest. An easy gauge: For any standing exercise, your torso will be bent forward less than 45 degrees as you perform the move.

**The main move:** Squat

**How to do it:** Hold a barbell with an overhand grip so that it rests comfortably on your upper back. Set your feet shoulder-width apart and keep your knees slightly bent, back straight, and eyes focused straight ahead. Slowly lower your body as if you are sitting back into a chair, keeping your back in its natural alignment and your lower legs nearly perpendicular to the floor. When your thighs are parallel to the floor, pause, then return to the starting position.

**Perfect it:** Arch your lower back and push your knees outward as you lower your body. "This keeps the stress off your knees and lower back, providing you with the safest way to perform the move," says Dave Tate, CSCS, powerlifting champion from Columbus, Ohio.

**Super substitutions:** Lunge, split squat, and overhead squat

## Movement 2

**Hip-dominant:** Any lower-body exercise in which your hamstrings and glutes work the hardest. For any standing exercise, your torso will be bent forward more than 45 degrees as you perform the move.

**The main move:** High stepup

**How to do it:** Use a step or bench that's 18 inches off the ground. Place your left foot on the step so that your knee is bent at 90 degrees. Your knee should not advance past the toes of your left foot. Push off with your left foot and bring your right foot onto the step, keeping your back straight. Now step down with the left foot, followed by the right. Alternate the leading foot, or do all of the repetitions leading with one foot and then alternating. Once you're comfortable, add dumbbells.

**Perfect it:** Use a knee-high step or box and hold a heavy dumbbell in the hand on the same side as your working leg, instead of two lighter dumbbells in each hand. "That ensures that the weight is focused directly on the target leg," says Cameron McGarr, CSCS. Using the combination of a knee-high box and heavy dumbbell will force your torso to bend forward, focusing the stress on your hips, hams, and glutes.

**Super substitutions:** Deadlift, Romanian deadlift, and back extension

## Movement 3

**Horizontal press:** Any upper-body exercise in which you push the weight out and away from your body

**The main move:** Barbell bench press

**How to do it:** Lie on your back on a flat bench with your feet on the floor. Grab the barbell with an overhand grip, your hands just beyond shoulder-width apart. Lift the barbell and hold it at arm's length over your chest. Slowly lower it to your chest. Pause, then push back to the starting position.

**Perfect it:** Try it with dumbbells. Start by holding the dumbbells next to your chest so that your palms face each other. As you push the weight up, rotate the dumbbells outward so that your palms are facing forward. "This works your pectorals the way they're designed to function, giving you better results," says McGarr.

**Super substitutions:** Pushup, dip, and close- or wide-grip versions of the barbell bench press

## Movement 4

**Horizontal pull:** Any upper-body exercise in which you pull the weight in to your torso

**The main move:** Barbell row

**How to do it:** Grab a barbell with an overhand grip and stand with your feet shoulder-width apart and your knees slightly bent. Let the barbell hang at arm's length on top of your thighs, thumbs pointed toward each other. Bending your elbows, lift your upper arms straight out to the sides and pull the barbell straight up until your upper arms are parallel to the floor and the bar is just below chin level. Pause, then return to the starting position.

**Perfect it:** Use a grip that's twice shoulder width and squeeze your shoulder blades together as you pull the weight to your chest. "You'll better work the muscles of your rear shoulders and upper back, which, when weak, cause men to slump and lead to the rounded-shoulder look," says Mejia.

**Super substitutions:** Dumbbell row, inverted row, and seated row

## Movement 5

**Vertical press:** Any upper-body exercise in which you press the weight upward

**The main move:** Barbell shoulder press

*(continued)*

# THE 20-MINUTE
# TOTAL-BODY WORKOUT (CONT.)

**How to do it:** Sitting on an exercise bench, hold the barbell at shoulder height with your hands shoulder-width apart. Press the weight straight overhead so that your arms are almost fully extended, hold for a count of one, then bring it down to the front of your shoulders. Repeat.

**Perfect it:** Hold the barbell with an "offset" grip, so that your thumbs are against the inside heads of the barbell. "This creates an imbalance in the distribution of the weight, forcing your shoulder muscles to work twice as hard," says Mejia.

**Super substitutions:** Barbell shoulder press and pike pushup

## Movement 6

**Vertical pull:** Any upper-body exercise in which you pull the weight downward

**The main move:** Lat pulldown

**How to do it:** Sitting on an exercise bench, grab a lat-pulldown bar with a "false" overhand grip that's just beyond shoulder width. A false grip means you place your thumb on top of the bar, alongside your index finger, instead of wrapping it around the bar. Pull the bar down to your chest. Pause, and slowly return to the starting position.

**Perfect it:** Perform the movement while on your knees instead of sitting on the bench. "It aligns your lats and your glutes, which naturally work together, allowing you to use more weight," says McGarr.

**Super substitutions:** Chinup and pullup

## IT STRENGTHENS BONES

As you age, you lose bone mass, increasing the likelihood that you'll one day suffer a debilitating fracture in your hips or vertebrae. That's even worse than it sounds, since Mayo Clinic researchers found that 30 percent of men die within 1 year of breaking a hip. In addition, significant bone loss in your spine can result in perpetually rounded shoulders and dowager's hump, eventually transforming you into a 21st-century Quasimodo. Resistance training can help you avoid this fate. Recent research in the *Journal of Applied Physiology* found that men who lifted weights for 16 weeks increased their hip-bone density by 3.8 percent and raised their blood levels of osteocalcin (a marker of bone growth) by 19 percent.

## YOU'LL GET MORE YEARS OUT OF YOUR OLD JEANS

A study in the *American Journal of Clinical Nutrition* found that for every pound of muscle a man loses, he gains a pound of fat. In other words, that 5 pounds of muscle that most men lose by age 50 is typically replaced by 5 pounds of fat. Not only does that make you look flabby, but it also increases your pants size, even if your scale weight remains the same. "One pound of fat takes up 18 percent more space on your body than 1 pound of muscle," says Dr. Volek. Bottom line: Keep your muscle, and you'll fend off fat.

## AND MAYBE TOUCH YOUR TOES AGAIN

Between the ages of 30 and 70, flexibility decreases 20 to 50 percent, making it harder for your joints to move through their full range of motion. For example, if you can't squat down until the backs of your thighs touch your calves (most men can't), you have tight hip flexors, which limits movement at the knees, setting you up for injury. In a study published in the *International Journal of Sports Medicine*, researchers found that three full-body workouts a week for 16 weeks increased flexibility of the hips and shoulders by more than 30 percent and improved sit-and-reach test scores by 11 percent. So there's still hope that someday you may once again be able to touch your toes. Weights can get you there.

## IT NEGATES THE DANGER OF EATING POTATOES

Every time you eat fast-burning carbohydrates, such as white bread, rice, and potatoes, your level of insulin—a hormone that helps keep your blood sugar normal—rises dramatically. That's a problem because consistently elevated insulin increases your risk of diabetes and heart disease. But lifting can help: Researchers at the University of Massachusetts found that men who added two full-body weight workouts a week to their existing aerobic exercise program had insulin levels that were 25 percent lower after a meal that was high in carbohydrates than the levels of men who performed the same aerobic exercise program but didn't lift weights.

## YOU'LL KEEP MORE FAST-TWITCH MUSCLES

It's not just the quantity of the muscle you lose that's important to pay attention to but also the quality. Research shows that the aging process reduces the size of your fast-twitch muscle fibers by up to 50 percent but shrinks the size of slow-twitch fibers by less than 25 percent. That's significant because your fast-twitch fibers are the muscles largely responsible for generating strength and power (the key to peak sports performance when you're young) and helping you easily get out of a chair when you're old, says Alex Koch, PhD, exercise researcher at Truman State University.

## YOU'LL REV UP YOUR METABOLISM

Your body requires energy to digest food. So every time you eat, you actually burn some of the calories you've just consumed—typically 15 to 20 percent. However, researchers at the University of Nevada found that you will burn 73 percent more calories when you eat right after you lift weights. Even better, scientists in the Netherlands calculated that men who lifted weights two times a week for 18 weeks burned an average of 9 percent more calories a day than non-lifters did. That's enough for the average man to lose 25 pounds in a year without making any changes to his diet.

## WEIGHT LIFTING WILL MAKE YOU WHISTLE

In a 2004 study at the University of Alabama, researchers found that older men who performed three weight workouts a week for 6 months improved their scores on measures of confusion, tension, anger, and overall mood.

# EAT TO STAY YOUNG

**Never skip breakfast.** It's the most important meal of the day for building and maintaining muscle, says Jose Antonio, PhD, CEO of the International Society of Sports Nutrition. The longer you go without eating after you wake up, the longer your body remains in fasting mode, making it more likely that your muscle will be broken down and used for fuel. Eating as soon as possible after rising in the morning ensures that won't happen.

**Eat protein and carbohydrates after a workout.** After exercise, your muscles are primed to take in glucose and amino acids. Researchers at the University of Texas Medical Branch found that you can speed muscle growth by consuming 6 grams of essential amino acids (the building blocks of protein), or about the amount in 12 ounces of milk. Add carbohydrates to the equation, by drinking chocolate milk, and you will speed up muscle repair, says Dr. Antonio.

**Take a daily dose of creatine.** Exercise scientists at the University of Hawaii found that older men who took creatine increased muscle, strength, and power after just 7 days of supplementation. "Creatine is the single most effective supplement in existence, and it has no harmful side effects," says Dr. Antonio. One 5-gram serving per day will do the trick. We like Power Creatine from Champion Nutrition (www.champion-nutrition.com).

# RULES OF REPETITION

1. Twice a week, perform each movement of the 20-Minute Total-Body Workout in the order described on pages 34–36. In your first workout, do 4 to 6 reps of each movement. In your second workout, perform 10 to 12 reps of each movement. Alternating between these two repetition ranges during each session trains your muscles for both strength (the lower reps) and endurance (the higher reps).
2. Do the two lower-body movements as straight sets, performing both sets of Movement 1 (quad-dominant) before moving on to Movement 2 (hip-dominant). Rest 60 seconds between each set of each movement.
3. To save time, do Movement 3 and Movement 4 as a pair and Movement 5 and Movement 6 as a pair, resting 30 seconds between each set. That is, perform one set of Movement 3, rest 30 seconds, and then perform one set of Movement 4 and rest another 30 seconds. Repeat one time—for a total of two sets of each exercise—and then move on to Movement 5 and Movement 6.
4. Always rest at least a day or two between workouts.
5. Every 4 weeks, choose a new exercise from each movement category.

Although unsure of the mechanism, study author Gary Hunter, PhD, suggests, "It could simply be a feeling of accomplishment from having become fit and more confident in themselves." Makes sense: The study participants reversed a decade of age-related muscle loss and fat gain by adding 4 pounds of muscle and dropping 3 pounds of fat, while increasing strength by an average of 42 percent. Those results would improve anyone's mood.

# Star Power

Big stars are paid big money to look great. We give you
their secrets for free.

**by Scott Quill**

I've just thrown an 8-pound medicine ball at Usher's face.

Not because he pissed me off. He's pretty cool, actually. And it's no comment on his music, either. Anything that gets women moving the way "Yeah, Yeah, Yeah" does is a boon for all mankind. I heave the weight at him because of what I want to get back: his secret. For this 60-minute sweat session at the Beverly Hills Hotel gym, he's my trainer, and I'm absorbing heavyweight information along with the medicine-ball tosses.

Just look at where this guy's career is right now—11 million copies of his CD *Confessions* in circulation, his trim form being strobe-lit by flashbulbs at the Grammys and the Oscars. So I've got a rare opportunity to learn from a master at the peak of his game. If I weren't so psyched to meet the guy, I could veer across the line into envy.

See, celebrities inspire the deadliest sins. Beauties like Eva Longoria fuel our lust. And Hollywood alpha dogs—the ones who access those Longorias like so many carnal ATMs—earn our envy. We see these men's sculpted bodies, watch them flex across movie screens and stadium stages, and wonder just what it takes for a guy to look that great. Our typical macho scoff: "Hell, I'd look that good if I had a personal trainer holding my hand for 3-hour workouts and a nutritionist cooking perfect meals every day."

Guess what? You're right. Showbiz types have both the money and the time to hire the best trainers to forge the best bodies. (Having the V-shape gene doesn't hurt, either.) But if you're still feeling that envious burn, consider this: It's their job. Abs are an asset. Bigger pecs mean a bigger paycheck.

That's why we can learn so much from celebrities and their trainers. They generate results. If they don't, their careers suffer, as any number of sex-gods-turned-caricatures can attest. To stay in the public eye, you have to be worth watching, and who among us wouldn't like a few more admiring glances? With that theory in mind, we've tracked down big names with big muscles and handpicked the best secrets from their personal programs. And that's also why I'm doing cannonball throws with Usher the day after the Recording Academy tossed three Grammy statuettes at him.

We're sitting toe-to-toe, legs spread in Vs, launching that medicine ball at each other. When one of us catches it, he lowers his back to the floor, then fires back up to a sitting position and returns the throw. Brutal. "Watch your breathing," warns Usher. "When it's burning, you can't give up. You don't pay attention to pain. Just breathe through it."

He shows me some wild moves, including a snakelike variation of the pushup. (For those of you following along at home: Usher's legs were straight and spread wide, hips high, forehead hovering just above the floor. He swooped down so his body was flat and just above the floor, then came up into a cobra, all in a fluid motion. Not only did it look cool, it worked almost every muscle in his remarkable body.) We also did an intense 5-minute circuit of Arnold presses, V presses, modified lateral raises, and pushups—all part of a routine he's using to build a back as ripped as his trademark abs. He stretches for 10 minutes before and after every workout and employs a combination of Pilates, yoga, and massage to loosen himself up for dance moves. He boxes and break-dances for speed and agility, lifts and runs for strength and endurance.

And for his abs? He eats.

"If you eat clean, you get better results," he says, lifting his sweaty beater and flexing. "Seventy percent of ab work is what you eat."

At age 26, Usher is dialed in—using advice from his trainer, Cliff Boyce, to achieve the body a millennial music star requires and also to stay healthy as life's pace quickens. We've adapted his plan, plus those of the Pistons' Ben Wallace, actor/adventurer/seducer-of-fine-women Matthew McConaughey, and seven-time Tour de France winner Lance Armstrong, and we've added in a strength and conditioning plan from Mark Verstegen, whose programs have fortified professional athletes at his Arizona gym.

## USHER'S WORKOUT PLAN

Under the eye of his trainer, Cliff Boyce, Usher combines moves for body, mind, and voice. Here's a typical workout.

**Meditation and visualization:** 20 minutes
**Static stretching:** 10 to 15 minutes
**Intervals:** 30 minutes on a treadmill or bike
**Strength:** 60 minutes of supersets and circuits
**Abs:** 10-minute circuit
**Static stretching:** 10 to 15 minutes
**Steam-room intervals:** 5 minutes in steam, 5 minutes in a cold shower, 5 minutes in steam (The contrast of hot and cold stimulates bloodflow to help his muscles recover; the steam keeps his voice smooth and his skin toned.)

# USHER'S GREATEST HITS

These life principles work for him. They can work for you.

**Usher on work:** "Imagine working in a studio till 4 o'clock every morning. You sit on a couch and waste energy. You eat a million and one things. So we built a gym in the studio, where I go pump some iron with Cliff [Boyce, his trainer]. Everyone looks at us like we're crazy, but when I go back into that booth, I'm pumped."

**Usher on stress relief:** "My life is work, work, work, work, work. So, naturally I have to have some moment for myself at the end of the day. Most of the time, I'll add a workout because it's something I want to do for myself physically, or I'll go and read a book, meditate, or whatever it may be, just to keep myself sane."

**Usher on health:** "At the age of 18 or 19, I broke down a lot. I'd get colds, catch the flu, 'cause I just wasn't taking care of my body. I wasn't eating right. I wasn't taking vitamins. I wasn't sleeping, which I still don't do. That's part of my problem—not resting."

**Usher on fitness:** "If you take care of your body, it'll take care of you. The benefit obviously is that I'm protecting my body from being harmed. I did my best to prepare and condition my body over time. If I didn't do this, I'd look a mess because of the lifestyle I live. I mean, the moment you go off, you notice the difference. You move slower."

**Usher on looks:** "Part of the selling of an artist is how you present yourself. If you look the part, people will believe you."

In short, we took elements of all-star workouts and built them into a program any man can follow.

Try not to think of the body gods on the following pages as pampered celebs; think of them as men with moves you can steal. Their plans are now your plans. So get to work. They can lead you through all the basic requirements for a fit body, including flexibility, strength, size, agility, and nutrition. They're giving you a red-carpet program that will make you a little more visible in the only place that really matters: your own world.

## PRINCIPLES OF FLEXIBILITY

Stretching isn't enough. You need flexibility training—a way to grow stronger and more powerful while reducing your chance of being sidelined. For proof, let's go inside the Palace of Auburn Hills, home of the world-champion Detroit Pistons. Look at Ben Wallace, with his 240-pound, 6-foot-9-inch frame. The first physical virtue that pops to mind as you watch

Wallace smash against bodies for a rebound probably isn't astounding flexibility. But that's what gives him his edge.

"NBA basketball players lose 20 to 25 percent of their ankle flexibility throughout the year because of all the calf work they do," says Pistons head strength and conditioning coach Arnie Kander, PT. Runners, tennis players, and other guys who train their lower bodies lose ankle flexibility. "Your calves get tight from moving forward, and then you start bending everywhere else." That's when the injuries start—and why you see so many basketball players come down with ankle sprains by midseason, Kander says.

Building a flexible body starts with a warmup. The Pistons use movement-based, or dynamic, flexibility techniques before each workout, practice, and game, and these are the best type of flexibility drills for you, too, says Kander. Think of it as movement rehearsal for your workout. These moves help muscles contract faster and more forcefully—something you need when you train for strength and power. This dynamic flexibility routine from Kander is surprisingly easy, takes only a few minutes, and will enhance the rest of your workout.

**Stationary march:** Marching in place for 20 to 30 seconds prepares your nervous system for activity by refreshing basic motor patterns. Bring your knees up to 90-degree angles as you march, to loosen your hip flexors, glutes, and hamstrings. Make sure your body stays upright, your pelvis remains neutral, and your toes point straight ahead. You'll begin to improve the alignment of your running stride, which will make you bigger, stronger, and faster. "If you run with perfect technique, you optimize the number of muscle units that fire," says Kander. "If you do that all the time, you'll excite muscles to fire just through running, and your muscles will grow as a result."

**Butt kick:** After marching, stand with your feet hip-width apart and bend one knee to try to touch your heel to your butt. Do 10 to 15 butt kicks with each leg to loosen your hamstrings and quads.

**Ankle-squat progression:** This progression of ankle squats prepares you to run with perfect form, says Kander, because your stance changes from wide to narrow, as it does when you run. Stand with your feet hip-width apart and slowly lower your body by bending at your ankles. Lower yourself only as far as you can without bending at your waist. Your upper body and trunk should remain upright throughout the move. Push yourself back up and repeat the motion for 10 to 15 repetitions. "Most sports require about a 10 percent bend at the ankles," says Kander, so try to improve your ankle flexibility to 15 to 20 degrees with ankle squats.

After a set of 10 to 15 ankle squats, place your feet narrower than hip width and move one foot forward so your feet are staggered. Now do another 10 to 15 ankle squats. Finally, place one foot in front of the other but a few feet forward, as if you were standing on a tightrope. Bend your leading leg slightly and keep your back leg straight. Hold this position for 15 to 20 seconds, then repeat with your other leg forward. This stretches your calves, hip flexors, and iliotibial bands—the bands of tissue that extend from each thigh down over the knee and attach at the tibia. As holding this position becomes easier, incorporate upper-body movements while your lower body remains perfectly aligned. For instance, move your arms through a running motion or do chest presses with your arms.

**Jogging progression:** Jog in place for 15 to 20 seconds, then jog forward and backward within about 5 feet so that you jog out three or four steps, then back a few steps. Keep your body upright and continue to jog in this small space for about 30 seconds. The weight shift of moving forward and backward wakes up your tendons, says Kander.

You can do a portion of this warmup as your cooldown. Perform the moves even more slowly. Add traditional static stretches (stretch and hold) to help your muscles restore their full length, but don't lose your focus just because

# BUILD SHOULDERS LIKE BEN WALLACE

Ben Wallace, the Detroit Pistons' all-star center, embodies what it means to be truly strong. "Ben does lots of core work, lots of flexibility. He's the first guy in the Pistons' workout room and the last to leave," says Arnie Kander, PT, head strength and conditioning coach of the Pistons. Follow the team's best drills and exercises to improve your all-around fitness.

**Stability:** To strengthen your rotator cuffs, the all-important stabilizers of your shoulders, bend your right arm so that your forearm is nearly upright and your hand is near your shoulder and perpendicular to the floor, palm toward you; your elbow should be directly beneath your shoulder. Now extend your arm straight up.

Your elbow is going to tend to shift out, and your palm will want to rotate outward. Don't let it happen. "Good shooters can keep their elbows in and their wrists square," says Kander. Alternate arms and do 10 to 20 reps daily.

**Agility:** "Basketball's a game of change of direction," says Kander. Try this drill instead of basic up-and-down suicides: Place a cone on each baseline and free-throw line and at half-court. Run the length of the court, stopping at each cone and shuffling all the way around it before sprinting to the next cone. Continue this to the opposite baseline and back.

the workout's almost over. "The mistake people make in stretching is failing to realize the strength it takes to hold positions. They become passive and just drop into positions," says Kander. An effective cooldown lasts 4 to 5 minutes.

## PRINCIPLES OF SIZE AND STRENGTH

Let's move on to Athletes' Performance in Tempe, Arizona, for the reason most of us work out—bigger, stronger muscles. Athletes' Performance is the training ground for professional athletes of every sport, including all-pros like Chicago Cubs shortstop Nomar Garciaparra, along with household-names-in-training like Tampa Bay Devil Ray Carl Crawford. "These guys are built to perform at high speeds with high power, and they look unbelievable, too," says Mark Verstegen, MS, CSCS, owner of Athletes' Performance and *Men's Health*'s Muscle Guy. "People would think they spend a lot of time bodybuilding. But they don't. Everything they have is for go, not just for show."

Building a body to perform will give you the best results even if your only reason for training is to attract attention at the beach. The first step is to set up a resistance-training program, and there are many ways to do this. For instance, you might do total-body workouts, alternate between routines such as upper-body/lower-body, or work pairs of muscle groups together. That's why, throughout these pages, we've included cool exercises and great tips for many types of programs.

What follows is a new plan, courtesy of Verstegen, so you can scrap your current routine if it has stopped yielding the results you want. The first step is to train movements, not body parts. This allows you to do upper-body pushing movements like bench presses and lower-body pulling movements like Romanian deadlifts in the same workout and lower-body pushing exercises like squats along with upper-body pulling exercises like lat pulldowns in another workout.

You'll also notice that the workouts include some total-body rotational movements to attack muscles in all planes. Organizing your workout around pushing, pulling, and rotational movements involves a tremendous amount of muscle mass each session, so your body releases more muscle-building hormones, stimulating greater increases in strength and muscle mass while shedding body fat. This also allows you to do upper- and lower-body exercises as supersets—pairs of exercises done one after another without rest—so your muscles have more time to recover between sets. The result: "You'll be able to go harder on the next set, recruit more motor units, and become bigger and stronger at the same time, as opposed to just trying to get a pump on," says Verstegen.

# OUTRUN INJURIES LIKE MICHAEL VICK

Quarterback Michael Vick acted fast after his injury in a 2003 preseason game, and his quick rehab saved his career. Andrew Bishop, MD, team orthopedist for the Falcons, proposes these active isometric exercises to preserve muscle after an injury.

**Ankle injury:** Lie perpendicular to a wall with your legs straight and push the foot of your injured ankle against the wall. Hold the contraction for a count of 5, then relax. Repeat 100 times a day.

**Knee injury:** Lie on your back with your knees bent. Try to straighten your injured knee and press it against the floor so your quadriceps contracts. Do 50 to 100 reps; add a straight leg raise if it doesn't hurt.

**WEEKS 1–3:** In Verstegen's program, adapted from his book *Core Performance*, you'll change the focus of your training every 3 weeks. (Exercise scientists refer to this as periodization.) The first 3-week phase is your foundation period, a time to perform a variety of exercises that incorporate stability and balance so you learn the proper movement patterns and can get more out of these exercises when you increase weights later in the program. Perform one or two sets of 10 to 15 repetitions of the following exercises twice a week. Rest 30 seconds after each superset.

Superset: Dumbbell alternating bench press; Swiss-ball leg curl

Superset: Dumbbell single-arm, single-leg row; split squat

Circuit: Dumbbell split curl-to-press; pushup or Swiss-ball pushup; dumbbell pullover extension; Swiss-ball lateral roll

After 3 weeks of training, take a few days to train less intensely and change the stimulus on your body. Verstegen calls this the reload period. You might try yoga, do body-weight exercises, or, as you progress in your training, return to the balance and stability moves you used in the 3-week foundation period.

**WEEKS 4–6:** For your next 3-week block, which Verstegen calls the extensive phase, you'll focus on gaining size, strength, and endurance. Do three or four sets of 6 to 10 repetitions of each exercise and perform each workout once a week. Rest 30 seconds between supersets.

WORKOUT A

Superset: Bench press; Romanian deadlift

Superset: Split squat; pullup

Circuit: Cable single-arm rotational row; dumbbell split curl-to-press; dumbbell pullover extension

WORKOUT B

    Superset: Dumbbell alternating bench press; split squat

    Superset: Dumbbell single-arm, single-leg row; Swiss-ball leg curl

    Circuit: Cable lift; cable chop; dumbbell split curl-to-press

**WEEKS 7–9:** After you reload, focus on building strength and power for 3 weeks (the intensive phase). You'll start to see improvements in all the sports you play. Aim for four to six sets of 3 to 6 repetitions using heavier weights for the following exercises. (Do 10 to 12 repetitions of the Swiss-ball Russian twist, Swiss-ball plate crunch, and Swiss-ball lateral roll.) Do each workout twice a week, alternating between them. Rest for 60 seconds between supersets.

WORKOUT A

    Superset: Bench press plus plyometric pushup; weighted pullup (Do 3 plyo pushups after each set of bench presses, rest 60 seconds, do a set of weighted pullups, then rest 60 seconds and repeat.)

    Superset: Dumbbell pullover extension; dumbbell split curl-to-press

    Superset: Cable chop; cable lift

WORKOUT B

    Superset: Cable single-arm rotational row; Swiss-ball Russian twist

    Superset: Split squat plus split jump; Swiss-ball plate crunch (Do 3 split jumps after each set of 6 split squats, then immediately do the Swiss-ball plate crunch.)

    Superset: Dumbbell front squat-to-press; Swiss-ball lateral roll

    Superset: Romanian deadlift; Swiss-ball prone knee tuck

    After you reload, continue alternating back and forth between intensive and extensive phases—always reloading after each phase. (Think of the time off for reloading as an investment in future muscle.)

## EXERCISE DESCRIPTIONS

### DUMBBELL ALTERNATING BENCH PRESS

Lie faceup on a bench holding dumbbells at the outside edges of your shoulders, palms facing your thighs. Lift both dumbbells straight up over your chest. Keeping one arm straight, lower the other dumbbell, touch it to the outside of your shoulder, then push it back up. Repeat with the other arm.

### SWISS-BALL LEG CURL

Lie faceup on the floor, put your heels on the ball, pull your toes up toward your shins, and pull your shoulder blades back and down. Squeeze your glutes until your body is in a straight line from ankle to shoulder. Keeping your hips tall, pull your heels in toward your glutes. Let the ball roll back slowly as you straighten your legs, keeping your hips elevated.

## DUMBBELL SINGLE-ARM, SINGLE-LEG ROW

Stand on one leg, grasping a stable surface (such as a dumbbell rack) in front of you with one hand. Bend by dropping your chest and lifting the leg opposite your free hand to create a perfect T with your body. Grab a dumbbell with your free hand. Pull it to the side of your waist and then lower it. Perform the designated number of reps with one arm, then repeat with the opposite arm and leg.

## SPLIT SQUAT

Set a barbell across your shoulders or hold dumbbells at arm's length at your sides. Step out into a lunge. Lower your hips toward the floor by squatting back and down. Without letting your back knee touch the floor, return to the starting position by driving your weight back up with your front leg. Do the designated number of reps with that leg forward, then switch legs and repeat.

## DUMBBELL SPLIT CURL-TO-PRESS

Stand holding dumbbells at your sides. Rest one foot on a bench or sturdy step that's about midthigh height in front of you. Perform a biceps curl, rotating your palms so they're facing you. Then press the dumbbells over your head, finishing with your palms facing forward, in, or backward. Do all your reps, then put your opposite foot on the step for your next set.

## PUSHUP

Get on all fours with your abdomen tight, pushing your chest away from the floor as far as possible. Lower your chest to the floor, then drive your body up explosively. Your shoulders and hands should be fully extended so your body is as far off the floor as possible.

## SWISS-BALL PUSHUP

Get in the pushup position with your hands on the ball and your fingers pointed down the sides of the ball. With your belly button drawn in, lower yourself to where your chest barely grazes the ball. Control the ball as you push back up.

## DUMBBELL PULLOVER EXTENSION

Lie faceup on a bench holding dumbbells with straight arms over your chest or eyes. Keeping your upper arms in the same position, lower the dumbbells until your elbows are bent 90 degrees. Now lower your upper arms until they're parallel to the floor. Now pull your arms back to the starting position, straightening your elbows on the way up. (*Note:* If you have shoulder problems, just do the first half of the movement, bending your elbows and then straightening them.)

## SWISS-BALL LATERAL ROLL

Lie faceup with the ball between your shoulder blades, hips fully extended and knees bent to 90 degrees. Extend your arms straight out to the sides. There should be a straight line from your knees to your shoulders and another straight line from hand to hand. Tighten your glutes to keep your body in line. Keep your belly button drawn in. Roll across the ball, reaching as far to one side as possible, holding your arms parallel to the floor. Keep your hips lifted.

## BENCH PRESS

Lie faceup on the bench with your feet on the floor. Keep your shoulders and hips in contact with the bench throughout the exercise. Grasp the barbell with a grip that's just wider than shoulder width and hold it with straight arms over your shoulders. Breathe in, lowering the bar to the lower part of your chest. Drive the bar forcefully back to the starting position. Extend your arms and shoulders fully at the end of each rep.

## PLYOMETRIC PUSHUP

Assume the standard pushup position. Quickly lower yourself to the floor, then push back up with enough force that your hands leave the floor. Land and immediately go into the next repetition.

## ROMANIAN DEADLIFT

Grab a barbell with an overhand grip just wider than shoulder width. Set your feet hip-width apart, with your legs in a fixed position but not locked at the knees. Your shoulders should be back and down and your weight should be concentrated on the back half of your feet. Shift your hips back and lower the bar as far as you can while keeping your back straight. Fire your hamstrings and glutes as you return to an upright position.

## PULLUP

Grab a pullup bar with either an overhand or underhand grip. (If you have acess to a bar with handles, you can take a "neutral" grip, with palms facing each other.) Hanging from the bar, pull your shoulder blades back and down to lift your body up. Finish by pulling with your arms.

## CABLE SINGLE-ARM ROTATIONAL ROW

Attach a handle to the low pulley of a cable machine. Kneel perpendicular to the machine, with your right knee and left foot on the floor. Reach across your body with your right hand to grab the handle, turning your hips and shoulders to the machine. Now rotate your right shoulder back and pull the handle to your right hip (much like a dumbbell row). Do all your reps, then repeat with your left side.

## CABLE LIFT

Attach a handle to the low pulley of a cable machine. Kneel perpendicular to the machine, with your right knee and left foot on the floor. Grab the handle with your left hand and turn your shoulders perpendicular to the machine, keeping your chest up and abdomen tight. Pull the handle up toward your chest while turning your shoulders and continue the motion by pushing it up and away, above your right shoulder. Lower your hands back toward your chest as you turn back toward the machine. Do all your reps, then repeat with the opposite side.

# GET SOLID LIKE THE ROCK

Building a rock-solid body starts with a well-designed workout plan. At the foundation of The Rock's is change; he switches gears in his cardio and strength training every 3 weeks. "A lot of people fail because they don't change their workouts in a systematic manner," says The Rock's personal trainer, Billy Beck, NSCA-CPT. This means focusing on building strength for a few weeks (The Rock lifts more weight fewer times), then on gaining size for another few weeks (he'll do more reps with lighter weights).

Using this approach, The Rock built leaner, more defined muscle for several of his recent films. In his plan, he includes time-saving circuits like these from Beck.

Perform the exercises one after another without stopping, and rest 60 seconds before the next circuit. Hold the last contraction in each set (at the bottom of the pushup and pulldown and the top of the lateral raise) for 10 to 30 seconds to exhaust your muscles.

**Circuit 1:** Dumbbell chest fly, dumbbell bench press, pushup

**Circuit 2:** Bent-over lateral raise, upright row, lateral raise

**Circuit 3:** Single-arm rope pushdown, two-handed rope pushdown, pulldown drop sets (10 pulldowns, decrease the weight for the next 10 reps, then drop weight again for another 10)

## CABLE CHOP

Attach a handle to the high pulley of a cable machine. Sit on a Swiss ball, perpendicular to the machine. Rotate your shoulders and grab the handle with both hands. Now pull the handle to your chest as you rotate away from the machine, continuing the momentum by pushing the handle down and away. Do all your reps, then repeat with your opposite side.

## WEIGHTED PULLUP

Attach a weight plate or dumbbell to a belt and strap it around your waist. Grab a pullup bar with either an overhand or underhand grip. (If you have acess to a bar with handles, you can take a "neutral" grip, with palms facing each other.) Hanging from the bar, pull your shoulder blades back and down to lift your body up. Finish by pulling with your arms.

## SWISS-BALL RUSSIAN TWIST

Lie faceup with the ball between your shoulder blades, hips fully extended and knees bent to 90 degrees. With your shoulder blades back and down, extend your arms above your chest, either keeping your palms together or holding a weight plate. Keeping your hips lifted, turn your shoulders to the right so they're perpendicular to the floor while your hips stay horizontal. Twist back to the starting position and then to the other side.

## SPLIT JUMP

Take a large step forward, keeping your chest up, shoulder blades back and down, abs tight, and knees and toes pointed straight. Lower your hips toward the floor by squatting back and down until your back knee nearly touches the floor. Hold this position for 2 seconds, then explode up, using your hips and legs and throwing your arms up at the same time. Extend your front leg and land back in the same split-squat position.

## SWISS-BALL PLATE CRUNCH

Lie faceup on the ball, arching your entire torso over it. Try to keep your shoulder blades, back, and glutes in contact with the ball so that your abdominals are completely stretched. Hold a weight plate behind your head. Roll your hips and chest up at the same time while pulling your belly button in. Crunch from the top of your torso and then lower your hips and chest to the starting position.

## DUMBBELL FRONT SQUAT-TO-PRESS

Stand holding dumbbells at shoulder height, with your elbows resting on your hips, palms facing each other. Initiating the movement with your hips, squat back and down until the tops of your thighs are parallel to the floor. Explode out of your hips and quads, using that momentum to drive the weights off your shoulders and overhead. You should finish with straight legs and arms. Lower the dumbbells back to your shoulders, then drop back into a full squat and repeat.

## SWISS-BALL PRONE KNEE TUCK

Get in a pushup position with your shoulder blades extended forward and your shins on the ball. Pull your knees to your chest until your toes are on top of the ball. Return to the starting positon and repeat.

## PRINCIPLES OF NUTRITION

A trip to Colorado Springs reveals that it's time to change the way you eat, especially if you follow the same diet every day. "If you're on a static diet, you're taking in either too few or too many calories at times, or not enough nutrients to support your training," says Chris Carmichael, Lance Armstrong's coach. Carmichael manipulated both calories and nutrients on Armstrong's training for his record seventh Tour de France victory.

In 2001, Carmichael created a periodized nutrition plan to fuel Armstrong's training, and it's hard to argue with the results. "By matching his nutrition to his training goals, Lance can stay healthy year-round and reach a pinnacle at the Tour de France," says Carmichael, author of Food for Fitness.

There's probably a time of year when you'd like to look or perform your best, which is why you need a predetermined and changing nutrition plan. The chief rule of Carmichael's approach is to view food as fuel for training, not a hungry response to it. In other words, adjust the number of calories and the amounts of nutrients you eat in order to optimally fuel the type, amount, and intensity of your training.

For instance, reduce your calories by 10 to 15 percent on days when you don't exercise, and "focus on foods that are high in antioxidants and protein to help you recover, especially cold-water fish." Salmon, albacore tuna, and halibut fit the bill, Carmichael says.

This nutrition approach benefits both strength and endurance athletes, but the plan that follows is particularly useful if you do a lot of endurance training or play sports often. First, record everything you eat and drink for 3 days, then calculate the percentages of carbohydrates, protein, and fat. (Software from www.nutricounter.com does all the calculations for you.)

## TAKE HOME BRAD PITT'S SIX-PACK

Okay, he's an amazing-looking man. But not even amazing-looking men necessarily look good in a skirt. Still, that's what the wardrobe masters had planned for Brad Pitt in the 2004 film *Troy*, so that's what he trained for.

Pitt already held a key to adding muscle below the waist: a solid midsection. "When you engage your stomach, it's a source of strength and stability," says Pitt's trainer, Gregory Joujon-Roche, president of Holistic Fitness in Los Angeles. The squat builds your entire lower body, and the power to squat comes not only from your legs but also from your abs, he says. Try this core-strengthening routine from Joujon-Roche. It will help your abs and make your lower-body work more effective.

**Weighted decline situp:** Lie on a plank board or decline bench set at a 45-degree angle. Hook your feet under the pads and hold a weight plate across your chest. Lift your shoulder blades off the bench, pause, then slowly lower yourself. Perform 10 to 15 repetitions, then, without resting, proceed to the roundhouse kick. Perform five sets of this superset.

**Roundhouse kick:** Stand with a punching bag in front of you. Lift your leg as if stepping over a bench and rotate your hips so the laces of your shoe, not the side of your foot, strike the bag. Lift and rotate the heel of your opposite foot. Flex your obliques on impact—then slowly pull your leg back. Do 25 kicks with each leg.

**Swiss-ball reverse crunch:** Lie faceup on the edge of a bench with a Swiss ball hooked between your heels and hamstrings. Roll your pelvis off the bench and, maintaining the same knee angle, bring your knees toward your chest. Pause, then slowly lower the ball to the starting position. Perform five sets of 15 to 20 repetitions.

# EAT FOR ENERGY
# LIKE LANCE ARMSTRONG

What you eat before, during, and after a workout may be the most important foods you eat all day. "Your body relies on glycogen stores to provide energy to your muscles and brain," says Chris Carmichael, personal coach of seven-time Tour de France champion Lance Armstrong. Eating additional carbohydrates throughout a workout helps power you through your activity. Eating immediately after a workout helps you recover faster and delivers protein to your muscles to accelerate muscle building. Sports drinks and shakes are an easy way to take in the nutrients you need while keeping up fluid levels, Carmichael says.

Carmichael's plan has four phases: foundation, preparation, specialization, and transition. You'll peak in the third phase, so work backward from your goal to determine when to begin. For instance, to peak for the Marine Corps Marathon in October, you'd start the foundation in April.

**Foundation:** Focus on general fitness during these 4 months. Do moderate-intensity cardiovascular work to build your endurance. Aim for 2.5 to 3 grams of carbohydrates per pound of body weight every day and 0.5 to 0.6 gram of protein per pound. Your carb-to-protein-to-fat ratio should be approximately 65-13-22 percent.

**Preparation:** Go harder and longer for the next 2 to 3 months, focusing on strength, speed, and power. If you play a sport, practice exercises and drills that will enhance the skills you need. For instance, basketball players might include suicides and interval work on cardio days, plyometrics in weight workouts. Runners will mix in sprints and long runs. Eat the same percentages of carbs, protein, and fat as in the foundation period, but eat about 3 to 3.5 grams of carbs and 0.6 to 0.7 gram of protein per pound of body weight. You should eat about 15 percent more calories during this period.

**Specialization:** It's peak time. Spend fewer hours training, but train more intensely than ever. This is when you're involved most in your favorite activity. Increase your carbs to 4 to 4.5 grams per pound of body weight (about 70 percent of your total calories); aim for 0.8 to 0.9 gram of protein (about 14 percent of your calories); and reduce fat to about 16 percent of your calories.

**Transition:** Recover for 1 to 2 months, but instead of collapsing on the couch, try a new sport or train about 25 percent fewer hours than you did in the foundation period. Eat 2 to 2.5 grams of carbs per pound of body weight and bump protein to about 0.6 to 0.7 gram per pound of body weight and fat to 22 percent of your total calories. Now's the time to start daydreaming about your next triumph.

## PRINCIPLES OF AGILITY

We're back in Beverly Hills to learn how agility training can raise your game by helping your body react faster. "It causes different firing patterns in the muscle," says Gunnar Peterson, CSCS. "You may look like a geek in the gym, but at the end of the day, who cares? I don't." After all, even if the actors and athletes Peterson trains—and the list includes Matthew McConaughey, Pete Sampras, Jennifer Lopez, and Mary J. Blige—look a little silly doing his agility exercises, their bodies look amazing, and move even better, when they're through.

Building a strong, flexible foundation allows you to train for agility, speed, and quickness, but you still have to progress slowly and carefully. Try starting with lateral hops. You'll need a low hurdle or anything you can hop over, such as a small cone or pillow. Stand with both feet on one side of the hurdle. Lift your inside foot—the one closest to the hurdle—and push off your outside

## BALANCE YOURSELF LIKE MATTHEW MCCONAUGHEY

When Matthew McConaughey's not running over rocks and through streams to keep his muscles guessing and growing, he uses uneven stances and uneven loads in the gym.

Add instability at any time in your workout to improve your balance and to stay mentally and physically engaged. Here's a sample progression for a biceps curl, but you can adapt it to lend an unstable boost to almost any standing exercise. "Whatever you think you can do, start one or two levels back from that," says McConaughey's personal trainer, Gunnar Peterson, CSCS.

Instability progression:

1. Biceps curl in a chair with a back
2. Biceps curl seated on a bench with no back
3. Standing biceps curl
4. Standing biceps curl on a folded towel
5. Standing biceps curl on an Airex Pad or Fit Disc
6. Standing biceps curl on a Bosu Balance Trainer
7. Standing biceps curl on the flat, more unstable side of the Bosu

Once you've mastered that over the course of a number of workouts, progress through the standing moves above on one leg, then finally with a dumbbell in only one hand.

foot to propel yourself to the other side of the hurdle. Land on what was your inside foot. Hop back in the other direction and continue hopping from side to side for a total of 12 hops. Practice until you can do 24. If you knock over the object, set it up and finish the set without stopping. Your movements should be quick, and you should pull your knees up into a tuck immediately after your feet leave the floor.

Peterson likes to incorporate lateral hops as a superset with jumping rope. "It teaches your body to move equally well in different directions," Peterson says, "which is a necessary skill for a more agile body."

Next, try hopping forward over the hurdle, using the same technique as you did for lateral hops. Then use a shorter object and try hopping backward. It feels weird at first. Progress to jumping forward and backward off both feet so it's like a broad jump.

Hops are only one component of agility. Running ladder drills and other sprints, or shuttles, also improves your ability to change direction. To do any of this agility work, you need balance as well as strength. (Check out the introduction to unstable surface training in "Balance Yourself like Matthew McConaughey," on the facing page.)

# The Gym-Free Workout Plan

Five ways to get bigger and stronger—without setting foot in a gym

### by Cameron McGarr, CSCS

Few men believe it, but you don't need barbells, dumbbells, or machines to build muscle; in fact, weight-training equipment often inhibits the process. That's because it requires you to be in a specific location, which might explain why more men consider themselves runners than lifters. After all, running is the most accessible form of exercise—anywhere you go, there's your gym. But learn a little bit about physics and the same can hold true for your muscle workout.

Consider the pullup: It's the standard by which all body-weight exercises are measured. And even the most hard-core lifters will agree that there's no better muscle builder for the upper body—with or without weights. The reason for its effectiveness: It takes full advantage of the scientific laws of motion and leverage, placing your body in a position that forces your back and arms to lift your entire body weight. Call it applied science at its finest.

Now imagine if all body-weight exercises were as challenging as the pullup. You'd be able to build anywhere—at home, on the road, or even in a public park. Physical science makes it possible. So with that said, here are the Five Laws of Body-Weight Training.

## LAW #1: THE LONGER YOUR BODY, THE WEAKER YOU BECOME

**The science:** By increasing the distance between the point of force (your target muscles) and the end of the object you're trying to lift (your body), you decrease your mechanical advantage. Think of it this way: An empty barbell is easy to lift off the floor if you grab it in the middle. But try moving a few inches in one direction, and it instantly seems heavier—even though its weight hasn't changed. The same is true of your body: Lengthen it, and every exercise you do becomes harder.

**Apply it:** Raise your hands above your head—so your arms are straight and in line with your body—during a lunge, squat, crunch, or situp. If that's too hard, split the distance by placing your hands behind your head.

## LAW #2: THE FARTHER YOU MOVE, THE MORE MUSCLE YOU WORK

**The science:** In physics, "mechanical work" is equal to force (or weight) times distance. And since your muscles and bones function together as simple machines—they form class 1, 2, and 3 levers—the same formula applies to your body. It's the most basic of principles: Do more work, build more muscle. Of course, in a weight-free workout, you can't increase force (unless you gain weight). But you can boost your work output by moving a greater distance during each repetition.

**Apply it:** Each of the following three methods increases the distance your body has to travel from start to finish, increasing not only the total amount of work you do but also the amount of work you do in the most challenging portion of the exercise.

*Hard:* Move the floor farther away. For many body-weight exercises—lunges, pushups, situps—your range of motion ends at the floor. The solution: Try placing your front or back foot on a step when doing lunges; position your hands on books or your feet on a chair when doing pushups; and place a rolled-up towel under the arch in your lower back when doing situps.

*Harder:* Add on a quarter. From the starting position of a pushup, squat, or lunge, lower yourself into the down position. But instead of pushing your body all the way up, raise it only a quarter of the way. Then lower yourself again before pushing your body all the way up. That counts as 1 repetition.

*Hardest:* Try minirepetitions. Instead of pushing your body all the way up from the down position, do 5 smaller reps in which you raise and lower your body about an inch each time. After the 5th minirepetition for a pushup, for example, push yourself up till your arms are straight. That counts as 1 repetition.

## LAW #3: AS ELASTIC ENERGY DECREASES, MUSCLE INVOLVEMENT INCREASES

**The science:** When you lower your body during any exercise, you build up "elastic energy" in your muscles. Just like in a coiled spring, that elasticity allows you to "bounce" back to the starting position, reducing the work your muscles have to do. Eliminate the bounce, and you'll force your body to recruit more muscle fibers to get you moving again. How? Pause for 4 seconds in the down position of an exercise. That's the amount of time it takes to discharge all the elastic energy of a muscle.

**NUMBER OF MUSCLES IN A MAN'S BODY:** 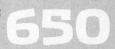 650

**Apply it:** Use the 4-second pause in any exercise. And give yourself an extra challenge by adding an explosive component, forcefully pushing your body off the floor—into the air as high as you can—during a pushup, lunge, or squat. Because you're generating maximum force without any help from elastic energy, you'll activate the greatest number of muscle fibers possible.

## LAW #4: MOVING IN TWO DIRECTIONS IS BETTER THAN MOVING IN ONE

**The science:** Human movement occurs on three different geometric planes:

- The sagittal plane, for front-to-back and up-and-down movements
- The frontal plane, for side-to-side movements
- The transverse plane, for rotational movements

Most weight-lifting movements—the bench press, squat, curl, lunge, and chinup, to name a few—are performed on the sagittal plane; the balance of exercises—for instance, the lateral lunge and side bend—occur almost entirely on the frontal plane. This means that most men rarely train their bodies on the transverse plane, despite using rotation constantly in everyday life, as well as in every sport. Case in point: walking. It's subtle, but your hips rotate with every step; in fact, watch a sprinter from behind and you'll see that his hips rotate almost 90 degrees. By adding a rotational component to any exercise, you'll automatically work more muscle—since you'll fully engage your core,

## PULL HERE FOR MUSCLE

The problem with body-weight exercises is that you miss out on pulling movements like rows, pullups, and curls. The answer isn't milk jugs and soup cans. For starters, a pullup bar is a great addition to any home gym—anything that's sturdy will get the job done. Unfortunately, a sturdy bar doesn't fit well in a carry-on bag, but that doesn't mean you have to miss your workout on the road. Try these solutions.

**JC Travel Bands:** Because these resistance bands are lightweight and attach securely to any door, they're perfect for travel. They're available in a variety of sizes for different strength levels. (about $20, www.performbetter.com)

**Blast Straps:** Loop these straps over a pullup bar, a ceiling joist, or even a jungle gym and you can perform suspended pushups, rows, and pullups. Because you "hang" from the bar like a gymnast, these straps add both rotation and instability to the movements, making them more challenging—and more effective. (about $55, www.elitefts.com)

as well as the original target muscles—and simultaneously build a better-performing body.

**Apply it:** Simply twist your torso to the right or left in exercises such as the lunge, situp, and pushup. (For an example, see the T pushup in Take 5, on page 69.) You also can rotate your hips during movements such as the reverse crunch.

## LAW #5: THE LESS CONTACT YOUR BODY HAS WITH THE FLOOR, THE MORE YOUR MUSCLES MUST COMPENSATE

**The science:** The smaller the percentage of an object's surface area that's touching a solid base, the less stable that object is. That's why SUVs are prone to rolling and tall transmission towers need guy wires. Fortunately, humans have a built-in stabilization system: muscles. And by forcing that internal support system to kick in—by making your body less stable—you'll make any exercise harder, while activating dozens more muscles.

**Apply it:** Hold one foot in the air during virtually any exercise, including pushups, squats, and deadlifts. You also can do pushups on your fingertips or your fists.

# S C I - G U Y

## Just Do It

Now there's research behind the Nike slogan. Successful exercisers don't think about having to train, they just get out there, says Sandra Cousins, EdD, exercise gerontologist at the University of Alberta. After conducting 40 interviews, she found that people who relied on self-pep talks to motivate themselves to exercise remained inactive. "They are simply not ready," she says. Need a jump start? According to a study in the *Journal of Sport & Exercise Physiology*, writing about your mortality can boost motivation. Write down how the thought of your own death makes you feel and read it in the morning. That should get you moving.

## Press Less

Do fewer sets for a bigger chest. In a new study published in the *Journal of Sports Medicine and Physical Fitness*, men who did fewer sets of bench presses with longer rest periods in between gained nearly twice as much strength as men who did more sets with shorter rest periods. Lifting the same amount of weight, the men did either four sets of 6 repetitions with 65 seconds of rest between sets or eight sets of 3 reps with 14 seconds' rest between sets. Fewer sets and longer rest periods "would appear superior for strength gains," says John Cronin, PhD, lead study author.

## Spin Off

Women in bike shorts, plus a great workout—do you need a third reason to take a spin class? How about this: A varied pace, like you'd get in a spin class,

**NUMBER OF MEN WHO'VE DROPPED A WEIGHT ON THEMSELVES:**

# 1 in 3

burns more calories than a steady pace, reports *Medicine & Science in Sports & Exercise*. In the study, 15 people did both a 30-minute spin session and a constant-rate workout. After the session, max $VO_2$ was greater among the spinners, leading to a 25 percent greater calorie burn. "For cyclists trying to lose weight, spinning classes can help you lose it faster," says study author Jie Kang, PhD, of the College of New Jersey. Try ending any workout with a sprint to raise your max $VO_2$.

## Monitor It

Your heart rate is a reliable gauge of workout intensity and fitness. So measure it correctly—with a heart-rate monitor. Taking your pulse with your fingers after exercise greatly underestimates your heart rate, according to the *Scandinavian Journal of Medicine and Science in Sports*. Study subjects who took their pulses at the wrist and neck 15 seconds after treadmill runs underestimated rates by 27 beats per minute (bpm) for low-intensity runs and by 20 bpm at higher intensities. Their hearts slowed quickly after the run, says study author Hirofumi Tanaka, PhD. Instead, use a monitor like Polar's F11 (about $160, www.polarusa.com). It has a comfy chest strap and won't pick up interference from other monitors.

## Be Patient

According to a new study by researchers at Arkansas State University, the oft-recommended 48 hours of rest between workouts may not be enough. After doing three to six sets of leg presses, 67 percent of the men studied needed 96 hours for their leg strength to fully recover. "The next question that needs to be addressed is, 'Do you have to be completely recovered to lift again and see gains?'" says Brian Church, PhD, the study's lead author. Until researchers know for sure, Dr. Church suggests keeping a log of your total volume (sets × reps × weight lifted). If volume dips, take some time off to thoroughly recoup your strength.

**NUMBER OF DAYS PER WEEK THE AVERAGE GUY LIFTS WEIGHTS: 3**

## Stay Strong

Great news for men hard-pressed for time: Researchers at the University of New Brunswick found that seasoned lifters can maintain strength with one workout a week. In the study, men who stopped working out for 9 weeks lost significant amounts of strength, while those who reduced their training from 3 days a week to once a week maintained their strength. "Over that short period of time, once per week appears adequate to maintain strength," says study author James Sexsmith, PhD.

## Tea Off

Green tea is approaching sainthood. Here's the latest miracle, verified by a study published by the American Physiological Society: Drinking green tea boosts exercise endurance. Japanese researchers supplemented the diets of mice with green-tea extract and tested how long the mice were able to swim (who knew?) until exhaustion. By the end of the 10-week study, the mice on the supplements improved their endurance twice as much as their counterparts had. Tea helps muscles "process lipids and use fatty acids as an energy source," says Takatoshi Murase, PhD, study author. The mice also got stronger, thanks to improved fat-burning capabilities. You can approximate the rodents' intake with about 4 cups a day.

## Lose It

Overweight men who can keep up with skinny guys may be fooling themselves. The strongest predictor of cardiovascular-disease risk is fatness rather than aerobic fitness. University of Colorado researchers screened 135 healthy men for 18 heart-disease risk factors and found that body fat was associated with higher scores in all categories, independent of aerobic capacity. One-third of the participants were vigorous exercisers with a wide range of body fat. Of course, it's better to be fat and fit than fat and wheezy, but overweight men should still strive to lose pounds, says study author Demetra Christou, PhD, of the University of Colorado's department of integrative physiology.

## Sweat More

Just 3 hours a week of moderate aerobic exercise reduces depression by 47 percent—making it as effective as antidepressant drugs, say researchers at the

Cooper Institute in Colorado. Exercise acts on the neurotransmitters serotonin and norepinephrine, both implicated in depression. The exercise can be spread out over the week, says study author Andrea Dunn, PhD.

Need more encouragement? Three hours of vigorous exercise (such as running or swimming) per week reduces stroke risk by 26 percent, according to a study that tracked 47,721 Finnish adults over a 19-year period. Moderate exercisers (4 hours a week of walking, gardening, fishing, or the like) showed a 14 percent drop in total stroke risk, according to the study from Finland's National Public Health Institute.

## Beat Cancer

Men with prostate cancer can cut their risk of dying of it by 70 percent through vigorous exercise, according to research from Harvard. The study looked at more than 47,000 patients over 4 years. The benefit was found in men over 65 who exercised intensely for 3 hours a week. Researchers believe physical activity affects hormones that would otherwise enhance the cancer's growth.

Research from the Dana-Farber Cancer Institute, in Massachusetts, showed that exercise lowered a person's risk of dying of colon cancer by 35 percent in the 3 years following treatment. The benefit came after at least 1 hour of moderately paced walking 6 days a week.

# WHAT'S NEW

## Creamy Ibuprofen

TransDermal Systems, a Massachusetts company, has developed a cream-based delivery system for ibuprofen. In addition to eliminating the risk of stomach bleeding associated with long-term use of oral ibuprofen, a cream version of the pain reliever would greatly reduce the total amount of ibuprofen entering the body and allow people to target muscle pain more effectively. At the time of this writing, the company was preparing to submit the cream for FDA approval.

## Smart Shirt

Soon, coaches will know if you're really beat or just taking it easy. A new T-shirt has sensors sewn in that monitor how a body is working. The LifeShirt System, by a company called VivoMetrics, measures blood pressure, how much oxygen is entering the blood, the temperature of the core and skin, and respiration. The shirt, approved by the FDA, is now being used in research and may be publicly available within a year, for about $500.

## XTrainer

Cross an elliptical trainer with a recumbent bike and you get this mongrel—the SportsArt Fitness XTrainer, which SportsArt prefers to call a hybrid. The promise of a better workout without working harder sounds like snake oil until you sit and spin. Independent resistance systems keep your whole body engaged. Fingertip controls allow on-the-fly resistance changes, customized

**NUMBER OF PUSHUPS THE AVERAGE GUY CAN DO: 27**

training options, and heart-rate threshold control (www.sportsartfitness. com).

## Creatine Ethyl Ester

Have you heard? The buzz around gyms and GNCs is that a new supplement could supplant creatine monohydrate as the top muscle builder. It's called creatine ethyl ester, and it's supposed to outdo the original in several respects. Here's one claim: Because creatine ethyl ester is more water soluble, it can be absorbed faster and therefore be more readily available to muscles (5 minutes versus 2 hours). Another alleged edge: It can prevent the increase in water weight that often occurs with the classic formula. But is there scientific proof behind the sales pitch? "The hype is better than the research," says Richard Kreider, PhD, a sports-nutrition researcher at Baylor University. And, to date, that research has only been on rats. Stick with creatine monohydrate, but take it with 50 grams of carbohydrates and 50 grams of protein; UK researchers found that this combination makes creatine effective in nearly 100 percent of users.

## The Easy Whey

Most protein bars complete a workout by relentlessly exercising your jaws. But Hilmar Ingredients of California has developed a new type of whey protein hydrolysate (WPH) that results in protein bars that retain their pliability—and palatability. Researchers with the company use a special enzyme to produce the WPH, resulting in "softer" proteins. Bars containing WPH are already on the market. Look for WPH or hydrolyzed whey on the ingredient list, then squeeze the bar lightly to check for a soft texture.

# T A K E 5

## Sculpt Your Body

Five ways to build your body anywhere

Even if you're a longtime lifter, this body-weight workout will challenge you like never before. Skeptical? Put it to the test. Keep in mind that this is the most basic version. So if you find an exercise to be too easy, apply one of the Five Laws of Body-Weight Training, on pages 56 to 59. Perform the first two exercises as an alternating set. That is, do exercise 1, rest 60 seconds, then do exercise 2 and rest another 60 seconds. That's one alternating set. Do a total of three sets of each exercise. Next, do exercises 3 and 4 as an alternating set, following the same procedure. For the last exercise, do two sets and rest 60 seconds after each set.

### 1. BULGARIAN SPLIT SQUAT

Stand with your right foot on a chair behind you and your arms hanging at your sides. Keeping your torso upright, lower your body until your left thigh is at least parallel to the floor. Pause, then push yourself back up. Do 12 to 15 repetitions with each leg.

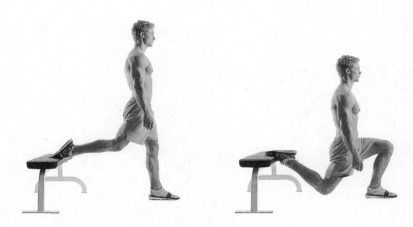

## 2. INVERTED SHOULDER PRESS

Get into the pushup position, but place your feet on a sturdy object that's about 2 feet high and push your hips up so your torso is nearly perpendicular to the floor. Bend your elbows to lower your head toward the floor. Pause, then press yourself back up. Do 8 to 10 repetitions.

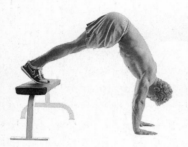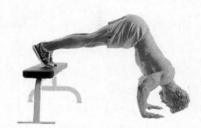

## 3. SINGLE-LEG DEADLIFT

Stand on your left foot with your right foot raised behind you, arms down in front of you. Allow your torso to lean slightly forward as you lower your body straight down until your hands touch the floor. Pause, then push back up to the starting position. Do 5 or 6 repetitions on each leg.

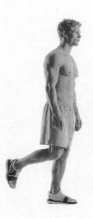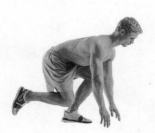

## 4. T PUSHUP

Lower your body as you would in a normal pushup, but as you push yourself up, lift one hand toward the ceiling and rotate your torso and hips in the same direction until you're facing sideways. Return to the starting position and repeat with your other arm. Do 10 to 15 reps to each side.

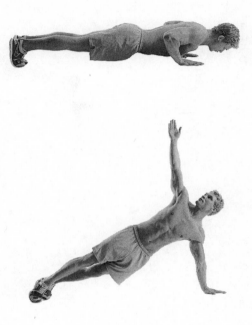

## 5. PLANK

Get in a modified pushup position with your forearms on the floor. Keep your abs tight and your body straight for 60 seconds.

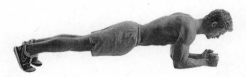

# MEN'S HEALTH
# QUIZ

## Will You Be Sidelined?

Take this test to find out if you're likely to be sitting the next one out

**1. Do you have a family history of knee or back problems?**
   A. No (0 points)
   B. Yes (+2)
   C. Yes, including surgery (+3)

**2. Do you snore?**
   A. No (0)
   B. Yes, but not very loud (+1)
   C. Like a jackhammer (+2)
   D. Not sure, but I feel rested (0)

**3. Do your shoes wear unevenly?**
   A. No. They're the same (0)
   B. There's a slight difference (+1)
   C. There's a big difference (+3)

**4. What's your body-mass index (BMI)? Calculate it at www.menshealth. com/BMI.**
   A. Lower than 25 (−2)
   B. 25 to 29.9 (−1)
   C. 30 to 32 (+3)
   D. Higher than 32 (+5)

**5. Have you ever smoked?**
   A. No (0)
   B. Yes, but I quit years ago (+2)
   C. I light up once in a while (+3)
   D. I smoke every single day (+5)

### 6. How often do you eat salmon or tuna?
A. Two or three times a week (−2)
B. A couple of times a month (+1)
C. Rarely (+3)
D. I eat some but also take a daily omega-3 supplement (−1)

### 7. Do you take a daily multivitamin?
A. Yes (−1)
B. When I remember (+1)
C. No (+2)

### 8. How often do you pop ibuprofen (Advil, Motrin) or naproxen (Aleve, Naprosyn) for muscle or joint pain?
A. Almost never (−1)
B. A few times a month (+1)
C. Daily (+4)

### 9. How many servings of dairy do you consume daily? (Eight ounces of milk, three or four small cheese cubes, or a 6-ounce container of yogurt each equals one serving.)
A. One (+2)
B. About three (0)
C. At least four (−2)
D. None (+4)

### 10. Do you regularly drink soda (either diet or regular)?
A. No (0)
B. Yes (+2)
C. Sure, but I stick with noncola varieties, like Sprite and 7-Up (+1)

### 11. How many hours do you usually sleep?
A. 6 to 8 (−2)
B. 5 (+1)
C. Less than 5 (+3)
D. More than 8 (+2)

### 12. How many hours straight do you spend sitting at a desk every day?
A. Less than 1 (0)
B. 1 to 2 (+1)
C. 2 to 4 (+2)
D. More than 4 (+3)

### 13. How often do you work out?
A. Three times a week (–4)
B. Once or twice a week (+1)
C. Monthly rather than weekly (+3)

### 14. Which workout plan most resembles your own?
A. Balanced blend of cardiovascular work, weight training, and stretching (–4)
B. Random mix of cardio and weight training (+2)
C. Either cardio or weight training exclusively (+3)

### 15. Do you feel stiff at the following times?
A. Upon awakening (that is, until showering or moving about) (+2)
B. After sitting still for a while (+1)
C. Only the day after a hard workout (+1)
D. Most of the day (+3)
E. I almost never feel stiff (–1)

*Test courtesy of Nicholas DiNubile, MD, orthopedic consultant for the Philadelphia 76ers. For the inside story on the science behind the test, go to www.drnick.com.*

## Rate Your Risk

**Zero or fewer points:** Almost invulnerable. You stretch without straining and bend without breaking. But don't get cocky—not even Cal Ripken Jr. was injury-proof.
**1 to 4 points:** Passably protected. There's a small chance you could be sidelined with a significant injury. Tend to those areas where you scored +1 or higher.
**5 to 12 points:** Inviting injury. The coin toss isn't for who gets the ball but whether this is the game when you go down. Overhaul your at-risk areas.
**13 or more points:** Walking wounded. Make an appointment with a certified physical therapist and bench yourself until what you learn from the PT lowers your score.

## Guard Your Target

**You score +1 or higher on 1, 3, 4:** Give extra attention to your knees.
**You score +1 or higher on 1, 2, 12, 15:** Give extra attention to your back.
**You score +1 or higher on 5, 6, 8, 11, 14:** Give extra attention to your muscle recovery.
**You score +1 or higher on 3, 4, 12:** Give extra attention to your lower body.
**You score +1 or higher on 5, 6, 7, 9, 10:** Give extra attention to your bone strength.

# BURNING QUESTIONS

## What's a good starter program for resistance training?

One of our most effective program strategies is what I call the A-B Split. Make two lists, one labeled A and the other B. Make sure every major muscle group is represented on one list or the other. Then assign an exercise to each muscle group. For example:

| A | B |
|---|---|
| Pecs: Dumbbell bench press | Lats: Chinup |
| Hamstrings: Leg curl | Quads: Stepup |
| Glutes: Lunges | Biceps: Barbell curl |
| Triceps: Triceps extension | Delts: Lateral raise |
| Traps: Barbell shrug | Calves: Calf raise |
| Abs: Reverse crunch | Lower back/glutes: Back extension |

You simply perform these workouts 3 days every week (Monday, Wednesday, Friday) in alternating order, starting with the A workout, then performing the B workout 2 days later, then going back to A, and so on.

The beauty of this arrangement is that you exercise each major muscle group three times every 2 weeks, a frequency we think is ideal. Then you'll need to change your list of exercises every 4 weeks to keep your body progressing.

## I do three 1-hour workouts a week. Will I get better results by doing six 30-minute workouts each week instead?

You will, for a number of reasons. Doing six short workouts versus three longer ones allows you to perform each exercise at a higher level of intensity before burning out. And by adding three workouts a week, you'll boost your metabolism that much more often. Here's a bonus: You'll end up eating less, too, since exercise is an appetite suppressant. If your schedule allows that much gym time, increasing the number of weekly sessions will pay off in greater strength and a leaner physique.

**When it comes to exercise, what the heck do *light*, *moderate*, and *vigorous* mean?**

Each describes a level of exercise intensity, says Carl Foster, PhD, director of the Human Performance Laboratory at the University of Wisconsin at La Crosse. Walking at your typical pace rates as light exercise, a jog that's tough but sustainable is moderate, and a full-out sprint is vigorous.

Still unsure if you're working hard or wimping out? Try the talk test. If you can sing while you're exercising, you're at light intensity. "If you do moderate exercise, you'll be in a range that just allows comfortable speech," says Dr. Foster. Practically speechless? You've entered the vigorous zone. Stay there for 20 minutes three times a week to meet Centers for Disease Control recommendations. Too chatty? Do 30 minutes of moderate exercise five times a week.

**Is it worse to skip exercise or get too little sleep?**

If you're short on time, it's healthier to get a full night's sleep and do a quicker workout every few days, says Jeffrey Gould, MD, sleep expert and clinical assistant professor of neurology at Temple University, Philadelphia, Pennsylvania. Chronic inadequate sleep can lead to high blood pressure, obesity, heart attack, and stroke, not to mention 100,000 or so car accidents per year. Best-case scenario: Hit the rack early so you can wake up in time for a full workout. If that's too much of a squeeze, sleep the full night and shorten your workouts—but up their intensity: less time between lifting sets, faster pace for cardio. You can hack it—after all, you'll be well rested.

**What's the best time of day to stretch?**

There is no best time of day to stretch, says *Men's Health* exercise-science advisor Steven Devor, PhD. The most important thing to remember is that it's always bad to stretch a cold muscle or muscle group. Elevate your heart rate slightly so the blood is flowing into the muscles that will be stretched. A warm muscle will respond more readily to the stretch and be far less likely to get injured.

**Is it possible to stretch too much? If so, how will I know?**

PERCENTAGE OF MEN WHO ALWAYS WARM UP BEFORE WORKING OUT OR PLAYING SPORTS: 43

## PERCENTAGE OF MEN WHO ALWAYS STRETCH AFTER WORKING OUT OR PLAYING SPORTS: 19

Anytime you feel a sharp or stinging pain, you're overstretching. Otherwise, it's not a concern. The consensus among most researchers is to hold a stretch for 30 to 60 seconds when muscles are warm, such as after a workout. Or try dynamic stretching beforehand; it's even more effective.

### Does alcohol slow muscle growth?

Yes. Alcohol virtually drowns testosterone, the key ingredient for muscle growth. "Just a single bender raises levels of muscle-wasting cortisol and increases the breakdown of testosterone for up to 24 hours," says Christian Finn, founder of www.thefactsaboutfitness.com.

### Is there a temperature at which it's just too cold to work out outside? I get tired of the treadmill.

If it's below freezing, dress in layers, with a moisture-wicking base layer underneath and a windproof shell on top. Below zero, we'd stick to a treadmill—the cold air can damage your trachea. A neoprene muffler can help warm the air if you really need to get outside. When you're finished exercising, go inside as soon as possible. As the sweat chills, your risk of hypothermia will skyrocket.

### What's the best liquid to use in a protein shake?

Milk. "Dairy products aid in fat loss," says Mary Ellen Camire, PhD, professor of food science and human nutrition at the University of Maine and a member of the *Men's Health* advisory board. If you're lactose intolerant, try the Lactaid or Dairy Ease brands, which can be found in most grocery stores. Use your shakes as a vessel to carry aboard the much-needed food group. You'll get the muscle-building power of protein along with fat-fighting calcium, while improving bone and cardiovascular health to boot.

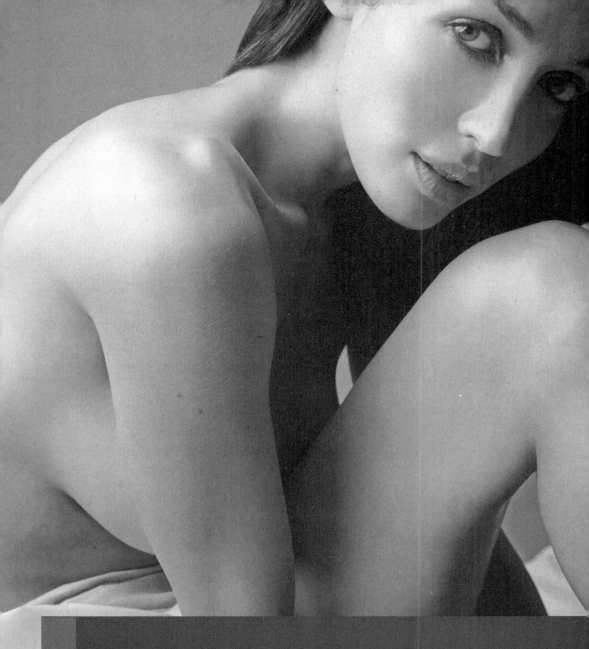

# THREE

# ENHANCE SEX

# READ UP ON IT

## Over the Top

Seven triggers to coax her to ecstasy

**by Nicole Beland**

**W**hen I'm this close to orgasm—eyes squeezed shut, lips twisted in a Billy Idol sneer, cheeks glowing—the most descriptive word wouldn't be *passionate* or *erotic*. It would be *determined*. Because right then, at the edges of my fading consciousness, I'm worried that the phone will ring, my knees will lose their traction on the sheets, or my boyfriend will change position, and suddenly I'll be sliding away from that elusive peak instead of moving toward it. For the 75 percent of women who don't always reach orgasm during intercourse, this happens all the time.

What we need is a fuse blower—that last shot of stimulation that blasts us into never-never land. "Calling it a fuse blower is pretty appropriate," says sex therapist Ian Kerner, PhD. "Recent studies show that in order for a woman to achieve orgasm, the part of her brain associated with stress, emotion, and anxiety has to shut down." If you're able to do something to a woman that feels so incredibly good that she completely relaxes and lets go, you're highly likely to make that woman climax.

My friends helped me compile this list of orgasm triggers. Get her to the point where she's sweaty and breathing fast, then try one.

### THE DOUBLE GRIP

Despite all the attention her booty may attract when she's walking down the street in tight jeans or bending over a file cabinet, a woman's butt is too

**AVERAGE AMOUNT A 24-YEAR-OLD MAN WILL DROP ON VALENTINE'S DAY: $157**

often sidelined during sex. And that's why grabbing both of her cheeks when she's on top may be just the unexpected turn-on a girl needs to get off. "The buttocks are packed with nerve endings," says Gilda Carle, PhD, a sex therapist in New York City. "To give her a surprising jolt of pleasure, spread your fingers wide and squeeze both buttocks firmly." But take it one step at a time. Yes, of course there are women out there who crave a good spanking, but until you've had a conversation about this sort of thing—however playful you are—just keep it simple.

## THE UP SHIFT

It was Rachel, my favorite sorority sister in college, who told me about this trick: "When a guy is on top of you in the missionary position, have him shift his body slightly forward so that, every time he thrusts, his penis rubs against your clitoris." Yes, Rachel really talked like this, and yes, college was fun. This tactic is even more orgasmic if the woman's legs are together and the man's are straddling her. "It increases clitoral stimulation," says Ellen Friedrichs, MA, an adjunct professor of human sexuality at Rutgers University. You can achieve the same effect when she's on top by propping yourself up on your elbows, which places your abdomen in closer contact with her sweet spot.

## THE ULTIMATE

There's no question that clitoral contact is the ultimate fuse blower. But how—and how much—depends on the woman. "Going down on a woman allows you to get a real sense of the stimulation she likes at every stage of arousal, especially the final one," says Dr. Kerner, who wrote a whole book on the subject: *She Comes First: The Thinking Man's Guide to Pleasuring a Woman*. It also eliminates any performance anxiety she has during intercourse, so she can kick back and enjoy. Learn what she likes. Get between her legs and give her a solid base of lips, tongue, gums, and even chin to rub against. At first, use your hands to guide her hips to let her know you want her to do the grinding. When she takes over, note how hard she's pushing and in what direction. Use that information later when using your fingers or giving her a more aggressive tongue bath.

## THE DROP TRICK

Steady clitoral contact is essential to female orgasm. But without adequate lubrication, it can become uncomfortable. "Lubrication increases the comfort and speed with which you can penetrate the vagina and grind against the clitoris," says Friedrichs. "But sometimes, no matter how turned on a woman might be psychologically, she can have trouble getting wet." Try a couple of drops of lube on the end of your tool. Then thrust with short, rhythmic strokes while pressing your body against her pubic mound. Don't use too much lube or it'll feel like throwing a hot dog down a hallway. Consider a pack of Astroglide "lubricant pillows" (www.condom.com). It's much nicer to pull an individual foil packet out of your bedside drawer than to use a sticky, half-empty tube.

## THE NECK WARMER

Our necks are highly responsive touch pads. The skin is thin and the blood vessels are close to the surface. Psychologically, it can remind some women of "their first sexual experiences, which could make it even more exciting," Friedrichs says. No hickeys, please: Don't suck. When you're having

# WHAT SHE'S THINKING...

We asked 400 women what they think about when fantasizing alone, on a scale of "Never" to "Almost Every Time."

|  | Never | Once or Twice | Once in a While | Frequently | Almost Every Time |
|---|---|---|---|---|---|
| Fantasy of what I'll do with my current partner | 7% | 8% | 21% | 44% | 20% |
| Rerun of a past encounter with a previous lover | 30% | 24% | 25% | 15% | 6% |
| Fantasy involving a celebrity | 38% | 31% | 18% | 9% | 4% |
| Fantasy involving someone I know and desire | 20% | 22% | 26% | 24% | 8% |
| Exhibitionist fantasy | 36% | 18% | 21% | 18% | 7% |
| Lesbian fantasy | 42% | 22% | 17% | 12% | 7% |
| Porn I've viewed in the past | 34% | 24% | 24% | 13% | 5% |
| Hot sex scene from a mainstream movie | 25% | 29% | 28% | 13% | 5% |

sex and she's clearly moving toward orgasm, brush your lips from her collar-bone to her jaw, then give her neck big, warm kisses until she comes unhinged.

## THE PLAY-BY-PLAY

For a verbal girl—and there are a lot of us out here—a string of four-letter words whispered in the heat of the moment can work wonders. "Start by complimenting her or talking about how good what you're doing feels," advises Friedrichs. If she doesn't say anything back, she might not be into it. If she responds with "Oh, yeah" or a similarly enthusiastic phrase, she wants more. "Nothing makes me hotter than when he describes what he's doing to me in explicit language," says my friend Lana. "But I'm picky—there are certain terms that drive me wild and others that make me cringe." Build a glossary: A goofy conversation over drinks about which anatomical nicknames are the sexiest isn't a bad idea. And if she ever seems horrified by what comes out of your mouth, just say, "Sorry about that, I got carried away." Final note: Skip cheerleader comments like "C'mon baby, you can do it!"

## THE DREAM MACHINE

"It's a simple fact that some women can climax only by using a vibrator," says Friedrichs. If your partner never hits her high note, no matter what you try, simply ask her if she's ever had a battery-assisted orgasm. If she says no, introduce her to a whole new world of wow by ordering something small but powerful, such as the Aqua Touch Vibe (www.goodvibes.com). If she's over the age of 30, her answer will probably be yes, and she'll be more than happy to pull her Hitachi Magic Wand out of her bedside drawer. After asking what pressure and speed she prefers (many vibrators have several settings), all you have to do is hold it against her clitoris as you move from one position to another. Enjoy the magic show.

# Hotter, Longer, Better Sex—Tonight

Three simple strategies to recharge your sex life

**by Bill Stieg**

Of course you wouldn't go to a sex therapist. Please. Everything's fine, everything works, everyone's happy. You'd like to get happy more frequently, sure, but you have no real complaints. And neither does the woman in your bed. Right?

You don't have to answer. According to our *Men's Health*/MSNBC poll, nearly half of American men aren't truly happy with their sex lives: 19 percent are "not at all satisfied," and 30 percent are a grudging "somewhat satisfied." And 43 percent call theirs "routine" or worse.

Let's admit it: We can all do better, for ourselves, our partners, or both— even if you're among the 3 percent who claim to get some every day. Quality counts, too, pal. But no, you don't have to go to a sex therapist. We've arranged for you to eavesdrop on some of the best. Give them 5 weeks and they'll give you a better sex life, one arousing step at a time. Take a peek.

## STEP 1: LEARN DENIAL

Bear with us. Denying yourself sex is the first step in "sensate focus," a form of therapy that sexperts say can help nearly everyone. It's often used for men who can't reach orgasm (they exist) and men who reach it too quickly (as many as one in three). But it can also work for couples who have lost interest in sex and those for whom it's become rote.

"It'll seem backward," says Michael Metz, PhD, a therapist in St. Paul, Minnesota. "But to find more pleasure, and to function better, you have to relax your body." So take your body off high alert. And that means...

**No porn.** You heard right. In the past decade, Dr. Metz says, Internet porn has caused bedroom trouble. A guy on the computer more than once a week, he says, is "more likely to be bored or not interested, to have erection

**NUMBER OF MUSCLES THE AVERAGE MAN USES DURING SEX: 143**

problems or trouble ejaculating. He could also have problems with PE [premature ejaculation]."

A week or two off can be enough. "Taking a holiday from porn can be good—it's like turning off the TV for a week," says Debby Herbenick, PhD, *Men's Health*'s "Bedroom Confidential" columnist. "Once you're not masturbating to porn, you're using your sexuality and mind and fantasies in a different way. And maybe you'll relate to your partner in a different way. Therapy often involves changing things up." Speaking of which . . .

**No sex.** Seems like you're already at this step? That's fine—these principles can work for couples across the frequency dial. In sensate-focus therapy, couples have bedroom sessions in which they take turns touching each other everywhere but the breasts and genitals. (They even start with clothes on.) In subsequent stages, usually over several weeks, they begin to include their fun bits in the touching—but still no intercourse.

For sexually dysfunctional couples, it's a way to rebuild from square one. For the rest of us, the steps—applied in 1 night—can be used to build excitement and rediscover the fun of the early days of sex. "They should do things that remind them of their first sexual experiences—over-the-shirt and over-the-panties touching," Dr. Herbenick says. "Just relive that for 30 minutes before diving in."

"People report that they have 'discovered' new ways of touching their partner, and enjoyed it, even when intercourse and orgasm are not on the agenda," says Cynthia Graham, PhD, a therapist and researcher with the Kinsey Institute. Further stages include guiding each other's hands, then touching at the same time, then the woman getting on top and rubbing before allowing penetration.

Try all the steps in 1 night—just incorporate that extra time. Take 10-minute turns touching and receiving—no genitals at first. Only after 20 minutes or so can you touch and receive at the same time. Relax and enjoy—anxiety causes the biggest problems. Ideally, you both stop worrying about performance and end up performing better than ever.

## STEP 2: TALK IT UP

So let's say you convince your girlfriend to go for a while just touching, and she doesn't dump you. In fact, she gets into it. She's guiding your hands where she wants them. She's giving back with her own creative touching and licking, and you're both reaching orgasm, often outside of intercourse. This is different; this is good.

## START TODAY

**What?** Sex with your clothes on.

**Where?** Perform a slow-mo grope on the couch when the kids have gone to bed. No kids? Do it with the drapes open. Sneaky is sexy. "Meshed in with the physical excitement is the excitement of knowing you could get caught," says Debby Herbenick, PhD, *Men's Health*'s "Bedroom Confidential" columnist.

**How?** Use fingers, feet, legs, tongues, whatever you can get away with to arouse each other. It's your white-hot teenage years all over again, when "you kept clothing on because you might have to put it back on really fast," Dr. Herbenick says.

**Why?** For many women (men, too), the sensations will be new all over again. "Do it just for the sake of variety," she says. "The breasts or genitals will feel different with fabric rubbing against them." Don't hold back. That's what doing laundry is for.

Bored couples have "lost communication—verbal or nonverbal," Dr. Herbenick says. It wasn't always that way. "Early in a relationship, there's more feedback. 'I like this. . . . Do more of that.'" Slowing down can bring this back.

**Make time.** "Scheduled sex is so underrated!" a fellow sex researcher blurted to Dr. Herbenick. "People say, 'Oh, come on,'" Dr. Herbenick says. But take 2 minutes to imagine how this could work.

For instance, she suggests that you call your wife on your cell on your way to work and formally request, "I'd like to make an appointment with Mrs. Whatever for 7:30 tonight," plowing right ahead, no matter how she reacts. Drop hints about what you're going to do; send follow-up e-mails with more hints and a countdown. "The whole idea of thinking about it really works. That kind of fantasizing is underrated, too," says Dr. Herbenick. "When you fantasize, you put the mind back into sex. It's integral to sexual enjoyment, performance, and orgasm."

**Exercise.** Drugs like Viagra relax the pelvic area to enhance bloodflow, Dr. Metz notes. You can produce similar results by tightening the pelvic muscles that stop urination and handle ejaculation. This trains the muscles and "helps you consciously identify the physical sensation of relaxing," which leads to better control and stronger orgasms, says Dr. Metz, the coauthor of *Coping with Premature Ejaculation*. "Hold it for 3 seconds, relax for 3 seconds," and do 10 repetitions (really), three times a day.

And go to the gym with your wife or girlfriend. It's known that physical fitness boosts libido. Now a new study from Duke University shows that losing just a little bit of weight makes both parties—women especially—more comfortable and enthusiastic in bed.

## STEP 3: HAVE FUN

Okay, you've slowed down your bedroom approach, learned how she—and you—like to be touched, and, by planning ahead, turned your BlackBerry into a sex toy. It's time to have some fun. "Your goal is to stimulate adrenaline, dopamine, and norepinephrine," says sex therapist and author Ian Kerner, PhD, "all those hormones that give you a high and lead to sexual arousal."

**Turn on (the TV).** Watch erotic videos together "as a warmup, to enrich lovemaking, not undermine it," Dr. Metz says. Give her the remote and tell her she can turn it off at any time, Dr. Herbenick says. She suggests veteran porn goddess Nina Hartley's interactive DVD *Sex Shooter,* which allows your partner to change the camera angle midscene—you may learn something about her preferences.

**Get slippery.** In your nightstand, store a lubricant that can double as massage oil, such as K-Y Touch Massage 2-in-1 (www.ky.com), and the book *101 Grrreat Quickies,* by Laura Corn, says Brian Zamboni, PhD, a sex therapist in Minnesota. Instructions for each quickie are in a sort of envelope that must be "unzipped"—good for shy couples.

**Keep it simple.** Cover her vulva with your hand and apply steady pressure to increase bloodflow. Everything you do afterward will feel better.

**Go slowly.** Don't make an expedition of finding her G-spot, and don't go too far or too fast. Insert a finger into her vagina no farther than your second knuckle. Wrap your finger around her pelvic bone and then slowly rock your hand until she starts to rock with you. Stay shallow, create a slow, throbbing sensation, and be gentle.

# The Final Frontier

An illuminating glimpse inside one woman's brain

**by Sarah Miller**

When you look into a woman's eyes, you probably often wonder, "What is she really thinking?" You truly believe that you want to know. Poor thing. Your curiosity is stronger than your fear. Very well, then. Every woman reacts differently, but my account here will scare the bejeezus out of you by coming pretty damn close to what your wife or girlfriend was thinking at various points in the arc of your relationship. Psychologists are standing by to help you understand—and deal with—us women. (You'll find their interjections here in parenthesis.)

## WHAT I WAS THINKING...THE NIGHT WE WERE INTRODUCED

Are you actually hot, or have I just made that up so I won't get bored and eat all this bread, which is awesome? I can't believe I have to be nice to your friend's girlfriend, who is phenomenally stupid, in case I want to date you.

(Women are acutely aware of the social network they may be joining, says Michael Cunningham, PhD, professor and psychologist. Men: Be nice to the entire group. Show that you'll work to make everyone at ease, says Diana Wiley, PhD, psychotherapist.)

Finally! You're looking at me. Chin's okay. Nice eyes, mouth...wait. Is your hair kind of gay?

(Look sharp. It takes less than 90 seconds for a woman to form her first impression, Dr. Wiley says.)

Oh. You looked away. I didn't like you anyway. I'm bored. I want more bread. Wow. You just totally smiled at me! If you hadn't, I would have just stopped talking to you, and you would have thought I didn't like you. But I wasn't going to be the one to stick my neck out, because that's your job. I wonder if your friend's girlfriend is going to be, like, a pain if I don't ask her to be in our wedding?

## WHAT I WAS THINKING...WHEN YOU PICKED ME UP FOR OUR FIRST DATE

Why aren't you here yet? My breasts look so good. But I'd better not catch you looking at them, because then I'll think that you think I'm easy. I have the greatest life! I am so pretty. You're 5 minutes late. I look like a total slut.

## NUMBER OF CALORIES SEX BURNS IN 20 MINUTES: 35

Where are you? You're 10 minutes late. I'm totally going to be a single mom.

(Females are extremely sensitive about their appearance and the possibility of rejection, says Dr. Cunningham.)

Oh, wow. Here you are. I am so crazy. You're cute. Like the suit—a little rumpled, neat but not trying too hard. If you want me to fall in love with you, you're going to have to do something about that hair. When I disappear briefly to get my jacket, I think I'll take off my underwear so I don't have panty lines. But I'd better put them in my bag in case you take me to a place that sells wings or jalapeño poppers. I'm classier than that, can't you tell? I'm already mad at you, imagining you taking me to a place like that.

(Know she's watching. Your clothes are a symbolic interpretation of you. She may think they reflect how you manage your money, how reliable you are, even what you're like in bed, says Patti Britton, PhD, sex coach.)

### WHAT I WAS THINKING ... ON OUR FIRST DATE

I blame you for my monologue in the car about my parents' dog's nail fungus. If you don't ask me a question in 5 seconds, we're not meant to be. Okay, 10 seconds. Fifteen. Ah, finally: "Do you like your job?" A little stiff, but you made the effort, and you are so lucky you said something before I reached 100.

Excellent restaurant choice—elegant but not stuffy. The hostess doesn't have our reservation. Great. Now you're going to freak out on her and embarrass me.... Oh, you just said, "No big deal. We'll get a drink at the bar while you work it out." I'm aroused by your restraint.

Wait a minute: You like the hostess! It was dark when we met. Did you remember me as younger, or blonder, or thinner? Like the hostess? I was lying when I thought I didn't want you to look at my breasts. Stop reviewing the wine list and look at them! I don't like you anyway.

I have to think of something flirtatious to say, to see if you respond favorably. Thank goodness I've only had one drink, so I'm still aware that "I'm not wearing any underwear" is not a good choice. Did you just say the wine list looks "approachable"? "Tell me you did not just say the wine list looks approachable." Whoa. Did I say that out loud? That was mean. Why do I have to be sarcastic when I'm feeling needy?

(Women have a sense of drama and want their partners to play their roles well, complete with witty repartee, says Dr. Cunningham.)

Oh, you're blushing and saying, "I'm just nervous because you're really pretty," and now you look embarrassed you said that. But trust me, it was the right thing to say.

(Another effective compliment: Tell her she's smart. Women love to hear this. She's worried about what she's not good at, so it's refreshing to hear what she is good at, says Dr. Wiley.)

We're such a good couple. It's totally cool if your friend's dumb girlfriend wants to be in the wedding. But she can't be a bridesmaid. She can do the guest book or something.

## WHAT I WAS THINKING...OUR FIRST KISS

I am putting my bare feet on the couch next to your legs. Wow. If you didn't get the memo on that one, you're past hope. Maybe you just don't even like me. I am making this really easy, dude. My toes are now touching your leg. Did you watch me walk to the kitchen and decide my ass is too fat and now you're trying to think of an excuse to leave?

(She's always bombarded by images of perfect women. Tell her she's beautiful, especially those parts women hate, to ease her insecurities, says Logan Levkoff, PhD, sexologist.)

Do I say something? No. My job is to wait for...wow, your hand is on my knee.

You're pulling me toward you. I am scared you have bad breath. Not too fast, very good, start off slow. I want to feel like you're dying to sleep with me but not like you're worried I won't. I can't believe I need everything to be perfect; it's going to be my undoing. I wonder if I'll date when I'm a single mom.

(Her perfectionism causes her to fixate on flaws and assume it means she'll be alone forever. This is called catastrophizing, which is more common in women than in men, says Dr. Cunningham.)

Closing my mouth a bit to slow you down worked. This is good. I should get one last thought in before I stop thinking, which is to remind myself to keep my underwear on. Oh. Right. Well, you can't touch where my underwear would be if I were wearing any.

## WHAT I WAS THINKING...OUR FIRST TIME IN BED

Should I put my legs up in the air, or is that too much? Why am I having sex with you? Oh...why not? I remember when I was younger and thought I was going to be a virgin when I got married. Now that is funny.

I am so glad I didn't eat any carbs or sugar for 3 days. My stomach is so flat! I like looking down at it while you're on top of me. It's so weird that I'm always thinking about getting married.

(Thoughts of marriage might be a way for her to justify having sex before she's ready, says Dr. Wiley. After sex, make a commitment to contact her. If you keep your word, her anxiety will abate, adds Dr. Britton.)

I wonder how many times I have to have sex with you before I can make you buy better sheets. I wish I were more like you. You don't seem to have a whole lot on your mind.

## WHAT I WAS THINKING...WHEN I ACCEPTED YOUR PROPOSAL

I am so in love. I am also relieved I'm not going to be a single mother. I hope I'm doing the right thing. I know why there is a giant ring associated with getting engaged, because every time I look at it, I feel enormously soothed.

(After this moment, reassure her that you love her. Do not stop trying to please her just because you popped the question, says Dr. Wiley.)

# SCI - GUY

## Get Some M&M-m-m-m-m-m-ms

Sex is like a box of chocolates: Even the disappointments are pretty good. A new Italian study of 163 women shows that those who regularly eat chocolate report enhanced sex drive and sexual satisfaction. The research left open the possibility that those who enjoy chocolate are just more sensual in general.

## Don't Kiss and Tell

Don't brag about your conquests. In a new study published in the journal *Sex Roles*, 8,000 people assessed fictional men and women who had varying numbers of sexual partners. Individuals—regardless of gender—were seen as less intelligent the more sex partners they had, suggesting that a double standard doesn't exist. Study author Michael Marks, PhD candidate, says people fall back on expected stereotypes ("sluts" and "studs") when talking in groups. But individually, they judge promiscuity harshly for both sexes.

## Admit It

Look around your office. If you were to marry a co-worker, who would it be? New research shows that men prefer an assistant for a long-term mate, though when it comes to one-night stands, they're equally eager to have one with a boss, peer, or assistant. In a study published in *Evolution and Human Behavior*, 120 men were presented with photos and hypothetical scenarios. The men rated their attraction to women of lower, equal, and higher workplace status. Results reflected caveman thinking: If we're dominant, we feel we can control her sexual behavior and ensure that our genes survive, says

**NUMBER OF MEN WHO'VE HAD SEX ON A BEACH:** **2 in 7**

study coauthor Brian Lewis, PhD, assistant professor of psychology at UCLA. A dominant woman is viewed as a reproductive risk because the man can't control her. (She might mate with that Neanderthal in sales!) The same study shows that women are not affected by a man's status in relation to their own.

## Enjoy an Added Bonus

In addition to saving your love life, the little blue pill may help heal your heart. Researchers at Virginia Commonwealth University found that Viagra prevents cell death after a heart attack. Credit goes to the drug's ability to boost nitric oxide levels in the blood.

## Quick Study

New research is helping to define premature ejaculation (PE). Nearly 1,600 men participated in a 4-week PE study in which each man's monogamous female partner held a stopwatch every time the couple had sex (talk about pressure) and measured how long sex lasted, from penetration to ejaculation. The 207 men diagnosed with PE went for an average of 3 minutes, compared with men in the non-PE group, who lasted for 9 minutes.

## Porn for Sperm

Scientists have discovered the kind of threesome that turns your sperm on, according to new findings published in the journal *Biology Letters*. In a study, 52 young men viewed sexually explicit images, then provided semen samples. The men who looked at images of two men and a woman had a higher percentage of motile sperm in their ejaculate, compared with men who viewed three women. The surge may be evolutionary, researchers speculate: The presence of other men means competition to fertilize an egg, so the sperm become livelier.

## Every Kiss Begins with $

If you're throwing money at a woman, spend it right. According to a British study, the best gifts in a serious courtship are extravagant but have no take-away value for her (to deter gold diggers)—for instance, expensive concert tickets or a weekend getaway, not rent money. Costly gestures indicate long-term intentions. From an evolutionary perspective, women are motivated to mate with men who are likely to stick around and help support babies. Dates that require considerable planning are also effective. Study coauthor Peter Sozou, PhD, says, "Anything that takes up a lot of a man's time—as long as the woman knows that—could be a signal of future commitment."

## Save Her with Sex

Keeping your wife happy can do more than prevent marital discord; it can also save her life. A recent study in the *Archives of Internal Medicine* found that happily married women are three times less likely to develop heart disease or suffer a stroke than are dissatisfied wives. Chronic stress caused by an unhappy marriage could be to blame, as it can cause high blood pressure and affect both cholesterol and blood-sugar levels.

## Speak Her Language

Men and women speak the same language after all. We're more alike in verbal skills than previously thought, according to a review of 46 studies conducted over the past 20 years. The idea that we communicate differently "is simply not true," says Janet Hyde, PhD, psychology professor in the Women's Studies Program at the University of Wisconsin at Madison.

## Clean Up

Can women sniff dominance? Czech researchers had 48 men wear underarm pads to collect body odor. Later, ovulating women smelled the pads and rated them. The most dominant men (determined by surveys) were rated most attractive. The preference may be a response to chemicals called androstenes, researchers say.

# WHAT'S NEW

## Moantone

The "vibrate" setting not doing it for you anymore? Now you can get a randy ring tone: Jenna Jameson and other porn stars will *ooh* and *aah* and utter unprintable phrases when you get a call on your cell. (See www.clubjenna.com for details.) We say keep this download on the down low. But it's your call.

## PE Drug

Researchers presenting at the American Urological Association's annual meeting reported that a new drug called dapoxetine, the first drug formulated to treat premature ejaculation, can help men lengthen intercourse. In a study of 2,614 men taking dapoxetine, participants saw a three- to fourfold increase in the amount of time between penetration and ejaculation. The FDA could approve the drug sometime in 2007. It's taken 1 to 3 hours before intercourse, and unlike other selective serotonin reuptake inhibitors, it acts fast and is cleared from the system quickly.

## STD-mail

You've got...a sexually transmitted disease (STD) notification in your inbox! A new Web site, www.inspotla.org, allows people to send anonymous or signed e-cards to casual sex partners they may have exposed to an STD, encouraging them to be tested. The site targets gay and bisexual men in the Los Angeles area, but anyone is welcome to use it. There's potential for misuse, admit program organizers, but a similar site in San Francisco has successfully prompted people to be tested.

**PERCENTAGE INCREASE SINCE 2001 OF YOUNGER MEN, AGES 18 TO 45, TAKING VIAGRA: 312**

## Viagra for Her

A new inhaled drug, developed by Palatin Technologies and known as PT-141, may be the woman's answer to Viagra. In a double-blind study, 8 out of 18 women suffering from sexual dysfunction reported such an increase in sexual desire and genital arousal after using the nasal spray that they had sexual intercourse that same day. Rather than enhancing genital bloodflow, PT-141 stimulates melanocyte receptors in the brain, which affect arousal. PT-141 is expected to hit the market in about 2010.

## Bar None

Massage oil in a bar gives new meaning to the term *spill-proof.* Ingredients in Lush Massage Bars include essential oils such as jasmine and bergamot, used by aromatherapists to enhance arousal. Smooth the bar on your hands as if lathering up or massage where you want to feel good. (www.lush.com)

# T A K E  5

## Supercharge Your Orgasms

Five steps to more satisfaction

When a man reaches orgasm, muscle tension and bloodflow to the pelvis peak, and the pubococcygeal muscle group, which supports the pelvic floor, spasms rhythmically at 0.8-second intervals. How can you possibly improve on that? Stronger contractions and more contractions, that's how. Stay away from non-FDA-approved supplements and herbal concoctions with outrageous claims. Follow these tips and you won't need any other help.

**Do Kegels.** Squeeze the muscle you use to stop yourself from peeing. Hold for a few seconds, then release. Repeat 20 times, one to three times a day. Another benefit of Kegels is that they can help with premature ejaculation.

**Find your plateau.** The plateau phase of sexual response is right before the point of "ejaculatory inevitability," when sex is often at its hottest. Be aware of your arousal levels. On a scale of 1 (nice jeans) to 10 (orgasm), try to keep yourself at a 7 or 8 and pause if you feel yourself losing control. This "peaking" will heighten the quality of orgasm because of the buildup of sexual tension and all those potent sex chemicals roiling in your system.

**Stimulate your P-spot.** The perineum is the smooth area between your testicles and anus. It's dense with nerve fibers and abuts the prostate. The prostate and perineal nerve fibers can be stimulated by pressing firmly against the perineum as you reach the point of no return.

**Make a ring.** Squeezing the veins on the side of the shaft restricts bloodflow from the penis. This creates tightness and pressure that boost the intensity of orgasm. Make a ring with your thumb and index finger and wrap it tightly around the base of your penis as you're reaching orgasm.

**Abstain.** Going without sex or masturbation will increase the volume of ejaculate and intensify orgasmic contractions.

# MEN'S HEALTH QUIZ

## Are You Getting the Sex You Deserve?

Take this test to find out if you're red-hot or not

**1. When you initiate sex, you're most like . . .**
   A. Babe Ruth: I strike out now and then, but I've hit a ton of home runs.
   B. Tom Brady: I complete every pass.
   C. The guy at the end of the bench: I get very little playing time.

The average guy has sex about twice a week if he's married—a little less often (once) if he's single, a little more (three times) if he's single but shacking up. If you're not hitting your number, work on your approach. In a University of New Orleans study, nearly 70 percent of men reported that when they initiate sex, they overestimate their partners' desire to get it on, most likely because they think women are like gas grills: Flick a switch and they get hot. Talking to her—about work, family, the news—is the greatest aphrodisiac for a woman because it establishes a bond of sharing that she equates with romance. To you, it's conversation. To her, it's intimacy.

**2. Your job most closely mirrors . . .**
   A. *Office Space*: same tasks over and over
   B. *Mission: Impossible*: dangerous
   C. *The West Wing*: stressful

You'd think stress would be as deflating to a sex life as a litter of puppies in the bedroom. But a stressful job (or even a dangerous one) involving some level of competition, as in law or sales, can actually improve it. "Real competition can drive up testosterone, which boosts libido," says Helen Fisher, PhD, author of *Why We Love*. "Being amped up by a high-powered, high-stress job is more likely to make you more sexually active" than idling in a cushy, low-key career. If work doesn't fire you up, seek a testosterone jolt in a recreational sports league. Men who get game increase testosterone levels by 15 percent, according to a Pennsylvania State University study. Even better, make her your steady doubles partner. The same study showed that women increased their libido-regulating testosterone by 49 percent during competition.

### 3. The most common sound to come from her mouth during sex is . . .
A. Laughter
B. A breathy moan
C. A stifled yawn

A Kinsey Institute study found that nearly one-quarter of women reported some distress in their sexual relationships in the preceding month. One of the most common causes of dissatisfaction: boredom. "The common denominator of satisfied couples is that they're very playful," says sex therapist Ava Cadell, PhD, author of *The Pocket Idiot's Guide to Oral Sex*. "My definition of sex is adult play. It should be fun and recreational. You should laugh and release all those pleasure endorphins. A sense of humor is an essential ingredient in great sex because it takes pressure off performance." Toys equal instant play. Shop together at a toy store (the kids' kind) for playthings you can bring into the bedroom. Imagine the possibilities with washable paint, masks, water pistols, and toy handcuffs.

### 4. On a typical night out, we . . .
A. Go to one of our two favorite restaurants and hit a movie afterward
B. Decide in the car
C. Our babysitter has too active a dating life for us to have one, too

The average man's sex life stays the same or even improves once he ties the knot. To ensure this outcome, do what good pitchers do—throw changeups into your nightlife at least once a week. "Novelty is good for sex, and I don't just mean novel sex. Novelty in your social life," Dr. Fisher says. It can be as simple as skipping dinner to play miniature golf or listening to a live band instead of the car radio. Anything that makes the start of your date less predictable can change up the ending, as well.

### 5. Quick: List all of your partner's pleasure points. How many did you come up with?

**PERCENTAGE OF MEN WHO SAY IT'S SMART TO CARRY CONDOMS: 77**

## PERCENTAGE OF MEN WHO ALWAYS CARRY CONDOMS: 23

A. Two or three
B. Five or six
C. Hold on, I'm still counting

A man should know at least 10 hot spots on his partner's body that drive her wild, says Dr. Cadell. Not knowing is a sign that you might not have enough colors on your palette to paint a sexual masterpiece. Simple technique—a kiss around the earlobe, a stroke between her toes—will help you find them. "Before you try to experiment with wild positions, be the best student of her body that you can be," says Gloria Brame, PhD, sex therapist and author. To find more spots, slow down your kissing, feeling, and touching so dramatically that it barely feels as if you're moving. "It's all about slowing sex down to find where she's receptive," Dr. Brame says.

**6. Your last compliment to her was about . . .**
   A. Her butt
   B. Her new shoes
   C. Her eyes

The way a woman feels about her body correlates with how inhibited she feels in bed. Sure, complimenting her shoes validates her taste, and saying something about her eyes reinforces her beauty. But praising her most guarded body parts—butt, thighs, waist—may be more important to your sexual satisfaction. "Women spend their lives trying to look good for men," Dr. Fisher says. "So a woman who feels she's sending the right visual signals is pleased with herself." The very best time for a "nice ass" shout-out is when there's absolutely no chance that you'll be having sex soon, like before you walk into her parents' house for Sunday brunch. "It's a gift to compliment her outside of the bedroom," says Dr. Fisher. Praising her body at times other than when there's a bulge in your pants reinforces your sincerity.

**7. How often does she have an orgasm during sex with you?**
   A. I've got her on a hair trigger
   B. Even Johnny Damon doesn't bat .400
   C. I have no idea

Only 30 percent of women can climax through intercourse alone; most also need direct clitoral stimulation, as evidenced by the fact that it takes women an average of 4 to 6 minutes to climax when they masturbate and 10 to 20 minutes during intercourse. "Making love with one's penis is like trying to write calligraphy with a thick Magic Marker," says Ian Kerner, PhD, clinical sexologist and author of *She Comes First: The Thinking Man's Guide to Pleasuring a Woman*. "The tongue is mightier than the sword." Assure your partner that going down on her turns you on and consider the virtue of the flat, still tongue, which she can move against to climax.

### 8. Our average sex session lasts . . .
A. 10 to 20 minutes
B. Three commercials
C. More than 30 minutes

The minimum duration of sex—including seduction, foreplay, and intercourse—should be about 30 minutes. "Anything under half an hour is not satisfying to a woman," Dr. Cadell says. If you're not quite there yet, build up your sexual stamina by aiming to make each sexual encounter a few minutes longer than the one before. Research shows that the average man lasts about 14 minutes during intercourse, but you don't necessarily have to go that long to satisfy her. For every 30 minutes of sex, only one-quarter to one-third of the time should be spent on actual intercourse, Dr. Cadell says. This leaves plenty of time for the other things she likes—decoupage!—and you won't feel as if you're being clocked.

### 9. How often do you have quickies?
A. Oops, I just did
B. Weekly
C. Rarely—she doesn't like them

Foreplay lasts an average of 12 minutes, and women would like it to go on for an average of about 18, according to a study by the University of New Brunswick in Canada. But that doesn't mean you can't take the express lane sometimes. One quickie a week is a significant sign that your relationship is strong—and that your partner understands your sexual needs, says Dr. Cadell. If she's nice enough to understand how much you need the 1-minute variety, reciprocate with the 1-hour kind (or at least the 18-minutes-of-foreplay kind).

### 10. How firm is your erect penis?
A. Granite

B. Garden hose

C. Linguine

You'd think erections would be like martinis—the stiffer the better. "The theory is that it should be rock hard, but if it's hard enough for penetration, it's probably okay," says Jon Pryor, MD, professor of urologic surgery at the University of Minnesota and a *Men's Health* advisor. The best time to do an erectile self-check is first thing in the morning—when the smooth muscle around the penis is relaxed, allowing blood to engorge it. If you wake up with a limp biscuit, it could be a sign of poor bloodflow or low testosterone.

## 11. What's your blood pressure?
A. Above 140/90 millimeters of mercury (mmHg)

B. Below 140/90 mmHg

C. No clue

"High blood pressure is an important cause of arteriosclerosis—and arterio-sclerosis blocking the arteries to the penis may be the most common cause of erectile dysfunction [ED]," says Thomas Lee, MD, a professor of medicine at the Harvard Medical School. Get your blood pressure checked at least once a year. Losing weight and exercising will lower your blood pressure as well as your body-mass index (BMI), another important number to know. (Calculate yours at www.menshealth.com/BMI.) In a 2003 Harvard study of more than 30,000 men, guys with a BMI over 28 had more than a 30 percent higher risk of ED than did men whose BMI was less than 23.

## 12. Does she know that you, uh, ring your own doorbell?
A. No. I tell her she's all I need.

B. Yes, but she pretends not to notice.

C. Yes. In fact, she helps.

"The more often people masturbate, the more often they have sex—it's a sur-prising correlation," says Dr. Fisher. "It's probably because sexual arousal ele-vates testosterone and dopamine, and that can lead to more sex." A woman who's cool with your self-pleasure—and who also masturbates—is likely to be a better lover because she knows what pleases her most, Dr. Brame says. A recent survey showed that 20 percent of women masturbate once a week and 60 per-cent of those women use sexual devices to do so. Need a last-minute Valentine's Day gift? The popular 4-inch Pocket Rocket (www.babeland.com) is discreet but packs a vibrating wallop. And the I Rub My Duckie vibrating bath toy (www.drugstore.com) makes showering together lots of good, dirty fun.

**13. If your fantasy is for you to play Justin to her Janet, you would . . .**
   A. Wallpaper her computer with the photo of their "wardrobe malfunction"
   B. Slip the idea into conversation between the meat loaf and mashed potatoes
   C. Buy a tear-away breast flap and nipple ring, and leave them under her pillow

Healthy couples share information on what they like and don't like. "You don't have to spend hours talking about your sex life," Dr. Brame says. "What's important is sharing with your partner something that's deeply intimate." Fisher suggests talking at a safe, nonsexual time. Women get intimacy just from talking, and this way, she won't feel pressured to perform right away—and that can make her more willing to put on the malfunctioning wardrobe another time.

**14. How old is she?**
   A. 20s
   B. 30s
   C. 40s

When men and women are younger, they tend to have more sex, but the quality increases with age. "As she gets older, she'll lose a lot of inhibitions and become more comfortable with her body," Dr. Brame says. "And that's probably the single most important thing in sex—feeling at home in your own body."

**15. What best describes what the two of you wear to bed?**
   A. Flannel
   B. Satin
   C. Flesh

Button-up pajamas send the message that she's not ready for sex. But sleeping in the nude doesn't necessarily indicate sexuality, either. The true green light: when she's giving some thought to what she wears—because that implies an element of seduction. Whether it's lace or a tight T-shirt, spending some time and thought preparing for bed is a sign that she's more open to sex. If she's a flannel gal, you can't quickly turn her into a garters-and-see-through-nightie fan. Start slowly: Buy her a pair of flannel boxers and a cotton tank top. She feels the comfort; you see some skin.

**16. When was the last time you had sex someplace other than the bedroom?**
   A. Last month

B. Last Saturday

C. Last girlfriend

"Don't always make love in the same place at the same time in the same position: It's the kiss of death in any relationship," Dr. Cadell says. In fact, you should always be striving to learn new techniques to satisfy her, like this one: Multitask while giving her oral sex. Lick her clitoris, stimulate her G-spot with one hand, and brush your other hand all through the intimate terrain of her butt. "If you can do that," Dr. Cadell says, "she's never going to let you go.

## The Scorecard

| | A | B | C |
|---|---|---|---|
| 1. | A = 2 | B = 3 | C = 1 |
| 2. | A = 1 | B = 2 | C = 3 |
| 3. | A = 3 | B = 2 | C = 1 |
| 4. | A = 2 | B = 3 | C = 1 |
| 5. | A = 1 | B = 2 | C = 3 |
| 6. | A = 3 | B = 1 | C = 2 |
| 7. | A = 3 | B = 2 | C = 1 |
| 8. | A = 2 | B = 1 | C = 3 |
| 9. | A = 2 | B = 3 | C = 1 |
| 10. | A = 3 | B = 2 | C = 1 |
| 11. | A = 2 | B = 3 | C = 1 |
| 12. | A = 1 | B = 2 | C = 3 |
| 13. | A = 2 | B = 3 | C = 1 |
| 14. | A = 1 | B = 3 | C = 2 |
| 15. | A = 1 | B = 3 | C = 2 |
| 16. | A = 2 | B = 3 | C = 1 |

**36 to 48 points:** Sack happy! (But then, you knew that.)

**22 to 35 points:** Bedroom for improvement.

(And stay in there until you get it right.)

**21 points or less:** Permafrost. Check Hot Spots, below,

for your personal danger zones.

## Hot Spots

**Seduction Skills:** Add your scores for questions 1, 4, 5, 6, 15, and 16.
10 points or less: You're no Colin Farrell. Poor scoring here means you
need to smooth out your game.

**Equipment:** Add your scores for questions 2, 10, and 11.

5 points or less: It's a poor workman who neglects his tools.

**Satisfaction: Hers:** Add your scores for questions 3, 7, 8, and 14.

7 points or less: Remember, fellas, there's a lady present.

Keep her happy and she'll reciprocate.

**Yours:** Add your scores for 9, 12, and 13.

5 points or less: Enjoy yourself, man.

Start by asking for what you want.

It'll help her open up, too.

# BURNING QUESTIONS

**Some days I want sex every 15 minutes. Other days I don't think about it. What gives?**

Chalk it up to your testosterone cycle. "Testosterone has daily, weekly, monthly, and yearly cycles. Men tend to be horniest in the morning, while weekly and monthly cycles are more individual," says Barbara Keesling, PhD, author of *Sexual Pleasure*. If your sex drive is stalling, your doctor can find possible causes, including low testosterone, medication side effects, or depression. Meanwhile, if you're feeling sluggish, order in. A study by the Smell and Taste Research Center in Chicago found that the smell of pizza can raise sex drive in men.

**Why is vacation sex always better? How can I have incredible, mind-blowing sex at home?**

Workday stress stimulates your sympathetic nervous system, meaning you're closer to ejaculation from the get-go. In women, it interferes with natural lubrication of the vagina. The bottom line: You have to cleanse your mental palate. Try hitting the gym, going for a jog, or listening to a CD. Then stretch out foreplay. More-relaxed sex means you'll have better gun control, and she'll be more likely to reach orgasm.

**How come women can have multiple orgasms, but men can't?**

You have a refractory period—the reloading phase during which men are unlikely to become erect or ejaculate again. It appears to be influenced by hormones, neurotransmitters, and nerve excitability and is seemingly absent among most women. It's unclear how many women can have multiple orgasms; research suggests that between 14 percent and 40 percent have experienced them. (And some women don't want to be pressured to be the next Energizer Bunny.) The closest thing to multiple orgasms for men is tantric sex, which often means learning to experience the sensation of orgasm repeatedly without ejaculating. Check out www.tantra.com.

### Why is it that whenever I'm not having sex regularly with my girlfriend, I feel depressed?

No surprise here: Sex makes you happy. Emotional and physical connections increase the brain's levels of serotonin, a natural mood booster. If travel is the problem, stay linked by doing something sweet for her while you're away. Or break out of your funk with a hard workout. Supersets might not be as fun as sex, but they'll help keep serotonin levels from bottoming out.

### Ever since my girlfriend started taking birth-control pills, she seems to want sex less often. Are they related?

Unfortunately, yes. The estrogen contained in most birth-control pills may lower levels of free testosterone, which is associated with libido. Others suggest that the blame may be misplaced, as sexual frequency tends to decline in long-term relationships anyway, Pill or no Pill. Desire and interest may also be influenced by stress, fatigue, depression, medications, and relationship issues. So, if she's willing, attack the problem on several fronts. Ask about lower-estrogen pills, hit the gym, and consider therapy appointments with either a psychologist or a sex therapist.

### I think having sex brings us closer. My wife disagrees. Who's right?

Both of you. See, women prefer feeling close first, then having sex. For guys, sex is pleasure first, then reassurance that the relationship is okay. So don't fight nature. Instead, use this knowledge to your advantage. Make her feel emotionally close to you with your clothes on. Women rely on words to connect. Increase the dialogue with her, and you'll enhance the odds of having more (and better) sex.

### Now that my wife is in her 30s, her sex drive varies wildly. What's going on?

Hormones. We're all a slave to them, but women become increasingly so as they progress through their 30s, especially with regard to testosterone. Women produce only about a 10th of the amount men do, but testosterone plays an equally important role in their libido, and it begins to wane in them after the age of 30. "Between the ages of 20 and 50, a woman's testosterone decreases by up to 50 percent," says Leah Millheiser Ettinger, MD, instructor of obstetrics and gynecology at Stanford University. "That can lead to a decline in sex drive." Short of suggesting hormone-replacement therapy—if you do, gas up the getaway car beforehand—there's nothing you can do about it.

The good news is that levels of testosterone and estrogen (also important in female libido) fluctuate over the course of a month, and by anticipating the highs, you can reap the sexual rewards. The first peak is 14 to 18 days into her cycle, during ovulation. A 2004 National Institute of Environmental Health Sciences study found that couples had 24 percent more sex during these days. The other peak time is during menstruation. But beware: Researchers at Charles University in Prague found that women are more likely to cheat during these days as well.

## Do those penis-enlargement creams and pills work?

Sorry, bud, you're out of luck. There are absolutely no data to support the use of any herbal product to boost penis size. Would-be enlargers like yohimbine, horny goat weed, *Cordyceps sinensis,* and tongkat ali may cause vasodilation, or enlargement of the veins. But that's just a short-term increase in erectile fullness.

## What's the safest brand of condoms?

Though all the condoms vetted in a Consumer Union test met preordained standards of toughness and durability, the Durex Extra Sensitive Lubricated Latex model withstood the most abuse. Planned Parenthood's condoms were the least durable. Although they met the standards for efficacy, they burst fastest when being filled with air.

## I've noticed I have cyclical mood swings. Is this a kind of male menstrual cycle?

While men certainly don't have menstrual cycles, most do experience mild or moderate mood swings. Fish oil, taken daily, has been found to help smooth out smaller attitude speed bumps. But serious mood disorders affect 7 percent of men. Some have a condition called cyclothymia, which causes significant changes in mood. And untreated bipolar disorder leads to extremes so severe that they can ruin your life. If your moods impair your ability to work, cause you to be inconsistent with your family, or rob you of joy, try therapy and possibly medication.

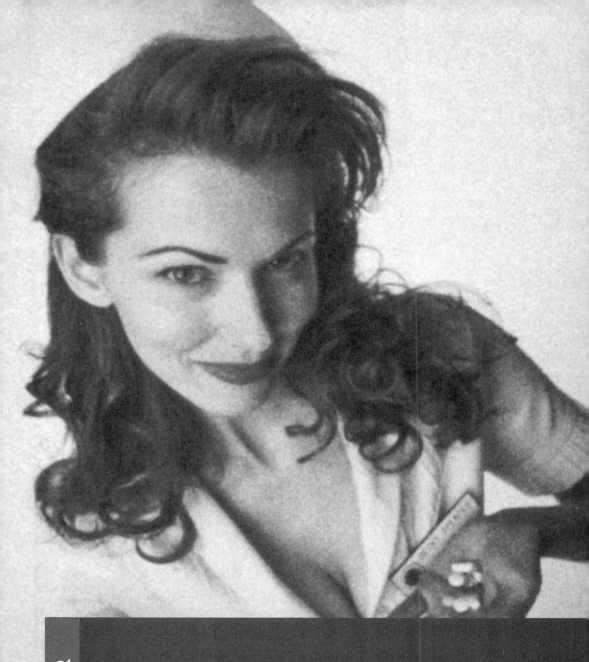

# FOUR

# STAY WELL

# READ UP ON IT

## Gut Check

Extinguish heartburn, eliminate ulcers, and solve other digestive
dilemmas with these easy steps

Dwight D. Eisenhower was a man with guts. He served as Supreme Allied
Commander to defeat the Nazis, strong-armed the Soviets in Geneva, and sat
in the Oval Office for two terms during the Cold War.

And yet, the one foe he wouldn't face was inflammatory bowel disease, a
condition that plagued him with stomach pain until finally, in 1956, Ike cried
uncle and underwent emergency surgery. Without the procedure, he would
have died. The lesson? Trusting your gut can save your life and ignoring it
could kill you.

Unfortunately, it's a lesson that millions of men still need to learn. "The
majority of the time, men will endure pain and irregular digestion, even vomiting, and think, This is just how I am," says Mark Lane Welton, MD, *Men's
Health* advisor and chief of colon and rectal surgery at Stanford University
Medical Center. The truth is, even though your body contains a food proces-
sor that rivals a Cuisinart, a lot can go wrong between the time dinner enters
your esophagus and the moment it exits your, well, you know.

So stop telling yourself nothing's wrong and start listening to your body's
digestive distress calls. Then read—and heed—our guide to beating the worst
gastrointestinal gremlins.

### HEARTBURN

Your body's food chute is your esophagus, a tunnel of muscle whose job
it is to push what you swallow into your stomach. And although this is supposed to be a one-way street, stomach acid sometimes rises back up, causing
the five-alarm fire we call heartburn.

Occasional heartburn can be caused simply by eating chocolate (it relaxes
the gatekeeping muscle known as the esophageal sphincter) or lying down
after a meal (the angle allows acid to escape). But a chronic burn can signal

gastroesophageal reflux disease (GERD), a condition that occurs when the sphincter stops working properly. Left untreated, GERD can lead to a worse esophageal ailment: cancer.

**Put out the grease fire.** A forkful of fat is as bad for your heartburn as it is for your heart. In a study published in the journal *Gut*, researchers surveyed 371 people about their eating habits and found that those who were heartburn-free ate 10 fewer grams of fat per day than the heartburn victims did. "Fats cause the lower part of the esophagus to relax, making it easier for the stomach to reflux," says Hashem B. El-Serag, PhD, lead study author. Eliminate 11 grams of saturated fat by ordering your morning latte with skim milk instead of whole and cut out 14 grams more by taking two of the yolks out of a three-egg omelet.

**Train your trunk.** When Norwegian researchers surveyed more than 74,000 adults, they discovered that those who exercised regularly had the lowest incidence of GERD.

In fact, the people who swam, jogged, or skied for 30 minutes once a week were 50 percent less likely to suffer from the condition than the couch potatoes were. The researchers speculate that as the diaphragm is strengthened by cardio training, it exerts pressure on the esophageal sphincter, preventing it from allowing acid to escape. And while any cardio exercise helps, according to Matt Fitzgerald, triathlon coach and author of *Runner's World Guide to Cross-Training*, freestyle swimming pushes the diaphragm's envelope like nothing else.

## ULCERS

Since acid is so damaging to your esophagus, you might wonder why it doesn't burn a hole through your stomach. One reason: a protective coating of mucus. But this barrier can be breached. Consuming copious amounts of coffee, overdoing it on ibuprofen and aspirin, and falling prey to the bacterium *Helicobacter pylori* can all wipe out mucus and allow acid to create ¼- to ½-inch holes, better known as ulcers, in your stomach.

**Do some navel gazing.** Is there a bug in your belly? Up to 90 percent of people with *H. pylori* don't know they're there, even though the bacteria may be wreaking havoc on their stomach lining, according to a German study that also evaluated the benefits of testing for the microbes. When the researchers screened 5,000 people for *H. pylori*—and offered treatment to those who tested positive—the incidence of ulcers plummeted by nearly two-thirds after 2 years. "Early treatment can prevent ulcers. If they start bleeding, they are fatal in 10 percent of cases," says Andreas Zober, MD, lead study author. "Among high-risk populations, *H. pylori* eradication can also prevent stomach cancer." Ask your doctor about having an ELISA test to detect levels of IgG antibodies against *H. pylori*.

**C the end of ulcers.** The best way to eat to beat *H. pylori* is to swallow more vitamin C. In a recent study published in the *Journal of the American College of Nutrition*, researchers measured the blood levels of vitamin C in more than 6,000 people and determined that those with the highest levels were the least likely to show evidence of *H. pylori* infection. Unfortunately, one of the best sources of C—orange juice—could aggravate an ulcer, thanks to its high acid content. So instead of ordinary OJ, pick up Tropicana's Low Acid formulation; one 8-ounce glass packs a day's supply of vitamin C, minus most of the acid.

## INFLAMMATORY BOWEL DISEASE

All in all, digestion is a pretty seamless process—unless you're one of the one million people with inflammatory bowel disease (IBD), a condition in which the lining of the intestines becomes inflamed. One theory suggests this happens because the immune system mistakes food for a foreign invader. White blood cells called T cells go wild and attack the intestinal wall, causing IBD sufferers to experience pain and diarrhea. And if IBD targets the large intestine, as it does in a form called colitis, the odds of developing colon cancer increase dramatically.

**Employ germ warfare.** Use yogurt to yank the rug out from under IBD. A recent study published in the journal *Gastroenterology* shows that treating IBD-afflicted intestinal tissue with probiotics—the good bacteria found in yogurt—encourages proper immune function. Plus, "probiotics limit bacterial invasion of the tissue," says Eyal Raz, PhD, lead study author. Next time you're in the dairy aisle, pick up Stonyfield Farm yogurt; it's the only U.S. brand that packs *Lactobacillus reuteri*, a strain of bacterium shown to act as an extra anti-inflammatory. Blend it with fruit to make smoothies or put a dollop on oatmeal.

PERCENTAGE OF PEOPLE WHO WASH THEIR HANDS AFTER SNEEZING OR COUGHING: 58

**Use slippery science.** Because IBD can raise the risk of colon cancer, don't hesitate to see your doctor if do-it-yourself treatments fail. New anti-adhesion medications can bind to white blood cells, such as T-lymphocytes, rendering them incapable of producing inflammation and damaging intestinal tissue. "It's kind of like putting Teflon on the T cells," says Matthew Grisham, PhD, professor in the department of molecular and cell physiology at the Louisiana State University Health Sciences Center. Ask your doctor about natalizumab (brand name Tysabri), a multiple sclerosis drug currently under FDA review for the treatment of IBD.

## COLON CANCER

Your large intestine is the gastrointestinal ground zero for colon cancer, the second leading cause of cancer deaths among men. Fortunately, colon cancer is unique in that screenings can catch its precursors, called polyps, long before they mushroom into something malignant. And the current gold standard of screening is the colonoscopy, a procedure in which a flexible, camera-tipped tube is inserted up the length of the colon. It's recommended that men go for a colonoscopy every 10 years, beginning at age 50.

**Put the freeze on franks.** Rule of thumb: If it comes in a bun, it could be catastrophic for your colon. In a recent study published in the *Journal of the American Medical Association*, researchers analyzed the eating habits of 150,000 adults over a decade and found that those who ate the most red and processed meats had a 50 percent higher risk of colon cancer than those who feasted on fish or fowl. Since the study didn't distinguish between lean steaks and fat-laden Big Macs, focus on cutting back on hot dogs, hamburgers (especially the fast-food kind), and sausages of every stripe. Instead, consume more chicken and fish, which contain nutrients such as selenium that may help ward off colon cancer.

**Dye to live.** Until recently, the best a man with a family history of colon cancer could do to offset his increased odds of developing the disease was go for a colonoscopy at age 40 instead of 50. Now there's a new lifesaving option: the high-magnification chromoscopic colonoscopy, a procedure that coats the colon with a dye designed to light up in the presence of precancerous cells. "It's able to go through the layers of the bowel, almost the same way an electron microscope would," says Dr. Welton. "This lets physicians remove suspicious cells before they develop into polyps." If colon cancer is in your genes, ask your doctor about a referral to a local cancer center or university hospital that offers the test.

# Warning Signals

Six minor health threats that could warn of major problems

**by Ted Spiker**

In most cases, men use a three-tiered system for handling medical problems: Gaping flesh wounds warrant a trip to the ER, blood-flecked phlegm calls for a doctor visit, and anything less demands a big dose of "suck it up."

And you know what? Sometimes this mentality makes sense, especially when so many minor conditions are merely inconveniences, the kind that can easily be cured with time, aspirin, or a sterilized Swiss army knife. That said, there are also instances in which ailments that seem innocuous—nosebleeds, knee pain, a new pimple—are actually harbingers of a heavy-duty health problem.

The key, of course, is knowing what's worthy of worry. We've made it simple. What follows is a brief rundown on third-tier complaints that just might be trying to warn you about a first-tier problem.

## BLIND SPOT: NOSEBLEED

We usually write off random nosebleeds because we think we know the cause—dry air, aggressive nose-blowing, angry ex-girlfriend. But out-of-the-blue bleeds can also be one of the few outward signs of high blood pressure, a condition that strikes nearly 8 percent of men between the ages of 20 and 34. If you don't have your blood pressure (BP) checked annually, your tip-off may come from a nasal gush. "You get nosebleeds because the small vessels in the nose have tiny cracks, and the high pressure pushes blood out of them," says Mehmet Oz, MD, professor of cardiac surgery at Columbia University.

If you can't connect your spontaneous spurt of blood to a specific trigger, make an appointment to have your BP checked (or pick up a Lifesource UA-787V home monitor and do it yourself). Anything between 120/80 and 139/89 spells prehypertension, while readings of 140/90 or higher indicate full-blown high blood pressure and the need for medication.

Whatever your score, try to begin every morning with oatmeal topped with flaxseed. A new study published in *Hypertension* showed that linolenic acid—a fatty acid found in flaxseed—is associated with lower rates of elevated blood pressure. And a study review published in the *Journal of Hypertension* determined that people who ate higher amounts of fiber dropped both their systolic and diastolic BPs by as much as 3 points.

## BLIND SPOT: SORE KNEES

It's not uncommon to feel a creak, tweak, or twinge in your knees after intense activity. But if the ache lasts longer than 2 hours, it may indicate osteoarthritis, says Virginia Kraus, MD, PhD, associate professor of medicine at Duke University Medical School. The first step, she says, is to rule out overexertion as the culprit. Cut back on the duration of your exercise regimen, then monitor your knee pain. "If symptoms persist beyond 3 months, it suggests an underlying musculoskeletal problem," says Dr. Kraus. (*Note:* If you had a knee injury when you were younger, you're especially prone to osteoarthritis, according to a Johns Hopkins study.)

The best way to ID osteoarthritis is with a standard x-ray, which will reveal whether the space between the joints has diminished due to cartilage loss. If the diagnosis comes back positive, talk to your doctor about acupuncture. University of Maryland researchers recently discovered that traditional Chinese acupuncture can decrease osteoarthritis pain by 40 percent. No joint trouble? Keep it that way by always icing your knees after exercise (the cold decreases swelling that sabotages cartilage) and by shedding about a dozen pounds. In a study review by the National Institutes of Health, people who lost 11 pounds cut their osteoarthritis risk in half.

## BLIND SPOT: SORE THROAT

Swallowing is sheer masochism when you have a sore throat, yet according to a recent study in the *Journal of the American Medical Association*, up to 40 percent of adults pop antibiotics for the condition, even though there's no evidence that the cause is bacterial. Most men, however, go to the other extreme and try to wait out a sore throat, no matter how much it hurts or for how long—not a wise move, especially if the sensation of crushed glass in your gullet lasts more than 3 days or changes the way you speak. Both symptoms signal the possibility of strep throat—and the need for professional help. "If the infection gets deep into your tonsils, the lymph nodes and surrounding tissue are overwhelmed with pus and can't drain," says Dr. Oz. "That can close your airways so you can't breathe."

Ask your doctor to swab your throat for a rapid antigen test, an exam that can detect a strep infection within minutes. If it comes back positive, then you really will need antibiotics. (Penicillin is still preferred.) On the other hand, a clean reading doesn't guarantee anything: The rapid antigen test is accurate only 88 percent of the time, according to a study in *Pediatrics*. Insist that your doctor send out your saliva sample for a bacterial culture, a strep test that's more time-consuming (1- to-2-day turnaround time) but more precise (95 percent accuracy). One other note: If your doctor is writing out a script for penicillin, ask him or her about adding one for the corticosteroid prednisone. Researchers in Israel recently found that sore-throat sufferers taking 60 milligrams of prednisone daily had 33 percent less pain after 12 hours than those who were given a placebo.

## BLIND SPOT: BLISTER

A blister caused by skin-on-sock friction may be a sign that you need to spring for new shoes, but it's hardly a health threat. However, blisters that pop up between your toes as a result of athlete's foot are, in fact, a medical emergency in the making. "When the blistering causes a crack between the toes, bacteria can invade the area," says Richard Braver, DPM, New Jersey sports podiatrist and fellow of the American College of Foot and Ankle Surgeons. "Every year, I have male patients who end up in the hospital for 5 to 7 days with IV antibiotics because of foot infections that could have been prevented."

That means intercepting the fungal infection before it reaches the blistering point. At the first sign of athlete's foot, do the obvious: Start using an over-the-counter cream such as Lamisil twice a day. But before your evening application, soak your feet in a solution of warm water and Epsom salts for 20 minutes; the salt will help suck moisture, a.k.a. fungus fuel, from the affected area. Follow this regimen for 2 weeks, and if you don't see improvement, ask your doctor about ciclopirox gel, a prescription medication that's been shown in studies to kick both fungal and bacterial butt. Already beset with blisters? Call your doctor; you may need antibiotics, stat.

## BLIND SPOT: PIMPLE

Acne is the Trojan horse of health. A bump that at first glance looks like a run-of-the-mill pimple may actually be basal-cell carcinoma, a slow-growing form of skin cancer. "Men as a group tend to ignore these lesions," says Edward McClay, MD, director of the San Diego Melanoma Research Center. So what's the difference between a zit and a tiny tumor? "The typical basal-cell carcinoma has a pearly appearance when light shines on it, and tiny blood vessels can be seen entering the nodule at the base," says Dr. McClay.

If you spot a pimple that won't go away, have a dermatologist check it out (and don't try to pop it—it could spread); basal-cell carcinoma is 95 percent treatable when caught early. The usual treatments—attacking it with a scalpel or using a combination of scraping and burning—can leave scarring, so consider getting zapped with a continuous-wave Nd:Yag laser. When researchers in Egypt treated 37 patients with this device, 36 were completely cured and had next to no scarring. The fact that one person in the study grew a new tumor isn't unexpected—the average recurrence rate of basal-cell carcinoma is nearly 25 percent—but it was avoidable. Everyone, especially cancer survivors, should not only slather on sunscreen (at least SPF 30) but also don sunglasses that provide 100 percent UV protection; a new Finnish study found that recent incidence of basal-cell carcinoma on eyelids has doubled.

## BLIND SPOT: LEG PAIN

It's easy to write off leg pain as a cramp, soreness, or the dog attached to your ankle. But it can also mean something's awry up top, in your heart. Here's why: The first sign of a gunked-up circulatory system is often leg pain, not chest pain, because the legs' longer blood vessels become blocked by plaque earlier, resulting in a shortage of oxygen to the muscles. And while that ache can occur anywhere below the waist—thighs, calves, feet—the "when" is often more specific. "Leg pain with arterial blockages usually gets worse as you exercise," says Dr. Oz, explaining that the greater the exercise intensity, the greater the oxygen demand.

The medical name for clogged leg vessels is peripheral artery disease (PAD), and one of the best tests for it is Doppler ultrasonography. If the ultrasound detects narrowed arteries and they don't pose an imminent threat, your doctor will probably prescribe exercise (taking breaks when the pain intensifies), a statin to lower LDL cholesterol, and a drug such as cilostazol to improve bloodflow. And the prescription for preventing PAD in the first place? Quit smoking, cut out all trans fats, drink more OJ to raise levels of HDL cholesterol (the good kind), and take 400 micrograms of folic acid daily. A study in the *Journal of Nutrition* found that men who swallowed supplemental folic acid every day had a 32 percent lower risk of PAD than those who didn't fortify themselves.

# Shut-Eye

Six tools for 8 hours of energy-boosting sleep

**by David Schipper**

Peter Powers puts people to sleep. He isn't boring; he's a hypnotist. In 1993, the Australian entertainer brought his trance-inducing act to Liverpool, where he made a man lie down in a shop-window display and fall sound asleep. Eight days later, the guy woke up (no doubt with a store-clearing case of morning breath).

Neat trick, huh? Unfortunately, unless you're sporting a gold pocket watch and excel at mind control (your own), this isn't something you can try at home. If you want amazing sack time, the kind that will boost your energy levels and slow the aging process, you need to build it from the bed up. That's why we tested a truckload of mattresses, sheets, blankets, and pillows to identify the ultimate combination for catching serious shut-eye. And for those occasional stare-at-the-ceiling emergencies, we also picked the best over-the-counter sleep supplement and prescription sleeping pill. Does all of this mean you'll snooze like the Liverpudlian? No, but you'll feel like you did.

## THE MATTRESS

There's more to take home from hotels than mini shampoo bottles. Chains such as Four Seasons, Westin, and W have been working with mattress manufacturers to create the most comfortable sleep surface possible. Made to the exact specifications of each hotel, the beds feature more coils and cushioning than even high-end store models. "It's the same reason hotels develop special blends of coffee," says Richard Adie, director of the Statler Hotel at the Cornell School of Hotel Administration. "Positive reactions mean return business." And, like the coffee, they're for sale. We tried five: the W Mattress, Westin's Heavenly Bed, Sheraton's Sweet Sleeper, the Four Seasons Signature Mattress, and the Four Points Four Comfort Bed. Although all were conk-out comfortable, only one was a sleeper hit.

**Best in class.** Thanks to a near-perfect balance of support and padding, the Four Comfort Bed (about $1,300 for king size, www.starwoodhotels.com) provides the ultimate slumber surface. The specially designed Sealy mattress sits atop a foundation made of heavy-gauge, high-carbon steel, which does a better job of flexing to absorb weight and movement than a traditional box spring. Need something softer? Check out the Heavenly Bed (about $1,450 for king size, www.westin.com); its pillow-top mattress provides an extra layer of padding that you can sink into without being swallowed up.

## THE SHEETS

If you shop for sheets, you'll come across the term *thread count*. This is marketing jargon for the number of threads woven into 1 square inch, the idea being that the higher the count, the softer the sheet. And that's true—up to a point. "You can't get more than 500 threads into a square inch," says Michael Breus, PhD, senior vice president at Phoenix Sleep LLC. "Companies will take two 500-thread-count sheets and weave them together and call it 1,000." Instead of looking for quadruple-digit counts, pay attention to the fabric. The rule: Go with natural fibers, such as cotton, and avoid synthetics, which are less absorbent, says Dr. Breus. "Over the course of an evening, you can release close to a half gallon of sweat and oils."

**Best in class.** Make your bed with Garnet Hill Signature flannel sheets (about $140 for king size, www.garnethill.com). A napped cotton surface makes these sheets somnolent soft. And, while warm, they weren't oppressively so. Runner-up: Pure Beech sateen sheets (about $100 for king size, www.bedbathandbeyond.com). They're woven with fiber from beech trees and were lighter than the Garnet Hill flannels and nearly as soft.

## THE BLANKET

Remember the best sleep of your life? Probably not, since it was when you were only hours old, says Gerard Lombardo, MD, director of the Sleep Disorders Center at New York Methodist Hospital. He says that one reason infants are born to sleep is because they're swaddled with blankets, which gives them the secure sensation of being in utero. So where does that leave an overtired adult? Shopping for a new cocoon. "Using a comforter can give you that feeling again," says Dr. Lombardo. Our mission: Crawl under a variety of fabrics filled with a range of insulations and discover which comforter is king.

**Best in class.** For that just-out-of-the-womb feeling, you can't beat the Isotonic Indulgence down-alternative comforter (about $200 for king size, www.bedbathandbeyond.com). It's filled with hypoallergenic synthetic-down fibers, which kept us warm but not baking the way goose down can. Of course, if you live in a hot zone, even the Isotonic may prove stifling. "If you're sweating, you're not going to sleep," says Dr. Lombardo. Go with Wamsutta's Egyptian cotton weave blanket (about $70 for king size, www.bedbathandbeyond.com); the weave allows cool air to circulate through.

## PERCENTAGE OF MEN WHO ADHERE TO LABEL RECOMMENDATIONS FOR OVER-THE-COUNTER PAIN-RELIEF DRUGS: 20

## THE PILLOW

If you're pillow-fighting with lingerie models, any old stuffed sack will do. But for sound, safe sleep, you need a pillow that will keep your neck aligned with your spine. "The more neutral your neck's position, the wider the nerve passageways running through it will open," says Mark McLaughlin, MD, spinal surgeon at University Medical Center at Princeton. The results: a reduced risk of neck pain and an increase in restful sleep. So what's the best prop for the job? Memory foam. "It's been a great advancement in pillow technology," says Dr. McLaughlin, explaining that memory foam molds to your head and neck, keeping everything lined up as if you were standing straight. And, unlike with feather fills, it won't lose its shape over time.

**Best in class.** Lay your noggin on the Select Comfort's GridZone pillow (about $90, www.selectcomfort.com). The egg-crate surface conformed perfectly to our tester's head and neck, dramatically reducing how much he tossed and turned. If you sleep on your back, though, the GridZone might be too thick. Try the Tempur-Pedic Classic (about $100, www.tempurpedic.com); it's a bit thinner, but still supportive.

## THE SUPPLEMENT

Despite its rep, melatonin isn't nature's knockout drug. "It's mostly effective in treating sleep loss related to your circadian clock," says Russell Rosenberg, PhD, director of the Northside Hospital Sleep Medicine Institute in Atlanta. So if you're lagging from a transatlantic flight or logging a 7-to-3 shift, pop a small dose of the hormone when you need to sack out (3 milligrams is plenty). But if all you want is a better, longer night's sleep, you'll need to swallow something else. We tried several supplements purported to provide quality shut-eye, then woke up and reviewed the research behind each.

**Best in class.** Only valerian root left us refreshed and had sound science to explain why. The root contains valerenic acid and valepotriates, two chemicals that have powerful sedative properties. In fact, a study in the *European*

*Journal of Medical Research* found that valerian is comparable to oxazepam, a medication sometimes used to treat insomnia. Look for the version from Nutrilite (about $25, www.nutrilite.com), which not only contains the most-studied formulation—450 milligrams, plus hops—but also, according to tests by Consumerlab.com, is free of contaminants.

## THE SLEEPING PILL

Popping a supermarket sleeping pill is a lot like whacking your head with a mallet: Both strategies will send you into la-la land, but it won't be a restful trip. "Over-the-counter products will change your sleep architecture," explains Gary Zammit, PhD, of the Sleep Disorders Institute at St. Luke's Hospital in New York City. In other words, over-the-counter sleep meds shorten the time you're in the deep stages of sleep, leaving you exhausted in the morning. What's more, the effects can last long after the alarm goes off and may make your head feel fuzzy. So if you try everything else and your sleep is still sub-par, talk to your doctor about a pharmaceutical fix. "Prescription pills are appropriate for both chronic and occasional insomnia," says Dr. Zammit.

**Best in class.** Ask your MD about Lunesta, a sleep drug that was approved by the FDA in late 2004. Unlike its chemical cousins Sonata and Ambien, which tend to lose their potency toward morning, Lunesta is effective throughout the sleep cycle—without disrupting the critical deep stages. It put our guinea pig to sleep in record time, kept him there for 8 hours, and left him feeling wide-eyed and alert the next day. And, according to Rosenberg, "your insomnia won't return twice as bad when you stop taking it," a common complaint about other prescription sleeping pills.

# S C I - G U Y

## Stress Less

Omega-3 fatty acids, also known as fish oil, are well-documented weapons against heart disease and stroke. But these good fats also help your body battle stress. A study published in *Diabetes and Metabolism* found that people taking 7.2 grams of fish oil a day for 3 weeks had significantly reduced reactions to stress. Get your daily dose (at least 2 grams is suggested) from a fish-oil pill like OmegaBrite.

## Beat Back Pain

Put away the pills and pull out the pocket watch. Hypnosis can relieve headaches and back pain, according to a study published in *Regional Anesthesia and Pain Medicine*. Researchers first determined the normal pain thresholds of 12 healthy volunteers, then hypnotized them. When the participants were given another dose of pain after hypnosis, 70 percent didn't feel it. Brain scans showed that hypnosis halted activity in the pain-sensing networks of the subjects' brains, says lead study author Sebastian Schulz-Stübner, MD, PhD. "Hypnosis can be used for all kinds of chronic pain, as well as for sedation and pain relief during minor procedures."

## Boost Your Immunity

Stop wasting sick days actually being sick. Conjugated linoleic acid (CLA) may give your immune system a boost. Scottish scientists gave 28 healthy volunteers 3 grams of CLA daily for 12 weeks and then measured their immune responses. The result: CLA elevated an important blood marker of immunity by 30 percent. "Supplementation could improve the body's ability to respond

NUMBER OF PEOPLE WHO SUFFER
FROM LOWER-BACK PAIN AT SOME POINT
IN LIFE: 4 out of 5

effectively to infectious agents and enhance resistance to allergens," says study author Klaus W. J. Wahle, PhD. For the best effect, divide your dose; in the study, people took two 500-milligram capsules with each meal.

## Say No to Drugs

If you're hacking up the proverbial lung, swallow cough medicine, not antibiotics. Antibiotics will not speed recovery from bronchitis, say British researchers. When they tracked 640 patients with bronchitis, they detected no difference in recovery time or symptom severity between those who took antibiotics and those who didn't. In addition to being a money waster, unnecessary antibiotic use can lead to the development of deadly strains of bacteria, says lead study author Paul Little, PhD. If you come down with bronchitis, stay home, get lots of rest, and wait a month before asking for antibiotics.

## Use the Right Jab

Heartburn? Pass on the Pepcid and try a Far Eastern fire extinguisher instead. Acupuncture may help stop heartburn, according to a new study. Acid reflux happens when the esophageal sphincter relaxes, allowing stomach acid to escape into the esophagus. Australian researchers found that using acupuncture to treat 14 heartburn sufferers tightened this control valve by 40 percent. Esophageal-sphincter problems may be stress related, says lead author Richard Holloway, PhD, which could be why acupuncture works. Go to www. acufinder.com to find a practitioner and have him or her focus on the Neiguan, a spot on the arm 2 inches above your palm.

## Crack One Open

First, eggs broke free of their artery-clogging reputation. Now, scientists have discovered a new reason to enjoy eggs: Eating eggs is one of the best ways to save your eyesight, thanks to lutein, a compound that's been shown to help prevent age-related macular degeneration. In a recent Tufts University study, researchers plied 10 men with lutein from eggs, spinach, and two supplements and then compared how well each source of lutein was absorbed into the bloodstream. Their finding: "The lutein in an egg is two to three times more bioavailable than that found in spinach or supplements," says study author Elizabeth Johnson, PhD. Double your potential return by eating eggs fortified with heart-healthy omega-3s.

# Hear This

Turns out the most advanced hearing aid may be the one you swallow. New research from Israel shows that vitamin E may help prevent—and even reverse—hearing loss. Researchers treated 66 people suffering from sudden hearing loss with either bed rest and steroid shots, or rest, shots, and 400 milligrams of vitamin E twice daily. Most of those who supplemented with E recovered 75 percent or more of their hearing, compared with just half of the people who received the standard treatment. Study author Arie Gordin, MD, reports that the vitamin may help repair oxidative damage that loud noises inflict on the delicate structures of the inner ear. There's still no cure for *Crossfire*, though.

# Back Talk Therapy

A bad back can put a man in a foul mood, and that mood can make the pain linger. New research suggests that treating depression helps heal chronic lower-back pain. In a study published in the *Lancet,* 400 lower-back-pain sufferers received physical therapy (PT) or were taught to manage pain with exercise and mental-health strategies. The latter group healed in the same amount of time as the PT group—with fewer treatment sessions. "Doctors need to find out whether patients' worries about their pain are keeping them from getting better," says lead study author Elaine Hay, MD. Ask your doc about stress-relief strategies before you sign up for weekly PT, she suggests. And do light exercise regularly. It can improve mood and strengthen core muscles crucial to back health.

# Pass on the Free Meds

Free can be a dirty word when what you're getting gratis is a handful of prescription drugs. Physicians who dispense free samples are more likely to prescribe pricey meds over generic versions, according to a study published in the *American Journal of Medicine*. Researchers studied 29 medical residents, half of whom agreed not to accept samples from pharmaceutical companies for 6 months. The doctors who still took handouts were 22 percent more likely than the abstaining MDs to prescribe name-brand drugs instead of cheaper, generic versions. If your doctor passes out free meds, ask whether this practice influences his or her prescribing decisions—and your pharmacy bill.

# WHAT'S NEW

## Smell Phone

Siemens is developing a microsensor that could detect changes in gases in the air. When implanted into a cell phone, it could "smell" blood-alcohol levels. No word on whether it will call a cab.

## Allergy Relief

Left loopy by allergy drugs? A new herbal supplement may work on hay fever without the groggy side effects. Researchers in India prescribed 1,320-milligram daily doses of Aller-7, a blend of herbs, plants, and black pepper, to 545 hay-fever sufferers for 12 weeks. More than 90 percent reported improvement in multiple symptoms. Aller-7 seems to control mast cells, which contain allergy-inducing chemicals. Find it at GNC outlets and www.drugstore.com.

## Message from the Bottle

Often if you forget to take a medication, you can forget about feeling better. But now, a new pill bottle, SIMpill, will text-message your cell phone when you forget to take your meds. Your pharmacist will program it when you pick up your prescription. For more information or to order SIMpill, log onto www.simpilldirect.com.

## Drill-Free Dentistry

Dental appointments may transform from torturous to tranquil. Japanese researchers are developing a paint-on synthetic enamel to fill cavities without

PERCENTAGE OF DOCTORS WHO DON'T WASH THEIR HANDS: **nearly 50** drilling. The compound, made of hydroxyapatite crystals and fluorine ions, will be brushed over the decayed area, where it will bond to enamel and halt the decay process. Studies are needed to ensure long-term safety before dentists can use it.

# Kinder, Gentler Alarm Clock

If waking up feels as if a giant adhesive bandage is being torn from your brain, you need a better alarm clock. This watch tracks your sleep patterns, identifies when you're nearest to consciousness, and gently coaxes you awake with a nonintrusive, if doggedly persistent, beeping. It seems to work most of the time, though sleeping with a watch on takes some getting used to (about $150, www.sleeptracker.com).

# T A K E 5

## Scratch That Itch

Five itchy problems, 10 simple solutions

How's your pruritus, pal? That's right—you, the one who just scratched his arm. And you, excavating your scalp. (There's treatment for that, you know.)

*Pruritus* means itching. And being a guy means scratching. Everyone itches, many times in many places, sometimes all over all at once. For such a common condition, however, doctors aren't exactly sure what's going on. Or why scratching feels so good. It's a tantalizing mystery, as unreachable as a mosquito bite in the middle of your back.

"I was attracted to the Zen nature of the symptom," says Jeffrey D. Bernhard, MD, dermatology professor at the University of Massachusetts and editor of *Itch: Mechanisms and Management of Pruritus*. "It's paradoxical: Dermatology is perhaps the most visual of all medical specialties, yet [in the case of pruritus] you can't see the most important symptom."

For ages, doctors and scientists thought itches traveled the same neural pathway as pain. That theory has recently changed. "We now know that itching has its own special pathway," says Adnan Nasir, MD, PhD, assistant clinical professor of dermatology at the University of North Carolina at Chapel Hill.

The sensation of itching is transmitted by tiny C-fiber nerves (the body's smallest) that extend nearly to the skin's surface. These C-fibers can be activated directly by an irritant that gets into your skin (through cracks) or indirectly by immune-system cells that patrol the skin and release histamine when they detect something foreign (such as mosquito spit). The histamine binds to the nerve endings, which send a message to the brain that the skin needs attention.

Pain uses a different set of C-fibers. "Pain causes a withdrawal response," Dr. Bernhard says. "Itching causes a response that makes you want to go toward the site of the itching."

Oh, does it ever. Why does scratching work, at least temporarily? "The brain can process only one signal of sensation at a time from a particular location in the skin," explains Dr. Nasir, "and by providing another type of irritation, we can suppress the itch." He also points out that scratching generates heat, "and if you heat up the nerves that cause itching, you can suppress it."

Which leaves the issue of why scratching feels so good. If you follow the "human urge to scratch, you're going along a well-trodden neurological pathway that is hardwired into the brain. It's very satisfying," Dr. Nasir says. Medicines or tricks (see below) that suppress itching are sometimes "not as gratifying." That shudder of pleasure may be from a "release of endorphins that give you a natural high," he says.

Too much scratching, however, can trigger an "itch-scratch cycle," in which the scratching aggravates the body into releasing more histamine, which causes swelling, which stimulates nerve endings, which causes more itching, and so on.

You need to break the cycle. We'll show you how, particularly with some classic male itches.

## DRY SKIN

Just because your skin isn't cracked like an old baseball mitt doesn't mean it's impermeable. Unseen irritants enter through unseen microscopic cracks, triggering inflammation, which aggravates the itch nerves. Compounding the problem, these cracks make it easier for moisture in the skin to evaporate. And the drier your skin, the more cracks you have, the more irritants sneak in, and the more agitated the itch nerves become. It's another one of those nasty cycles.

**Treat it.** You can't add much moisture to your skin, so trap it inside with the thickest moisturizer you can stand; thicker products create the best barrier.

## ALL-PURPOSE TRICKS

**Ice it.** Cold tends to make the C-fibers sluggish.

**Fool it.** Scratch the corresponding spot on the opposite limb. Nerves on one side of the body run up the other side of the spine and somehow "it tricks the brain," says Adnan Nasir, MD, PhD, assistant clinical professor of dermatology at the University of North Carolina at Chapel Hill.

**Ignore it.** Play a game on your Sony PSP to distract your brain. A recent Australian study published in *BMC Pediatrics* found that allowing kids to play a virtual-reality video game while they were being treated for burns resulted in reduced pain and itching.

Dr. Nasir suggests Aveeno Daily Moisturizing Lotion with Natural Colloidal Oatmeal. Not only is it light on extraneous ingredients that could cause allergic reactions in some people, but "the oatmeal binds to water, and some people think it has antibacterial properties as well," he says. Use it within 3 minutes of getting out of the shower; otherwise you won't be trapping anything.

**Prevent it.** Shower with lukewarm water, because hot water will "degrease your skin," eliminating natural oils that you need, says Jerome Litt, MD, assistant clinical professor of dermatology at Case Western Reserve University Medical School. But after you step out, crank up the hot water and turn off the bathroom's exhaust fan for a steam treatment while you shave. In fact, try to avoid dry air throughout your day; during the summer, turn off the air-conditioning every few days (it dries the air) and open the windows to let in humidity, suggests Dr. Litt. And if necessary, use a humidifier and set it for 55 percent relative humidity, the optimal setting for comfort. (Try the Holmes HM8405RC-U humidifier, which doesn't need a filter, has a base that can be washed in the dishwasher, and runs for 24 hours before needing to be refilled; about $30, www.holmesproducts.com.)

## ATHLETE'S FOOT AND JOCK ITCH

They're the same thing, actually; both are caused by the fungus *Tricho-phyton*. (The condition is called tinea cruris in the groin and tinea pedis on the feet.) And as most of us already know, this itch is a bitch to get rid of. "I've seen people with athlete's foot whom we've treated repeatedly without its getting better," says Dr. Nasir. "And then we found out they had jock itch as well. Once we treated that, the athlete's foot went away." Turns out they had been cross-contaminating themselves.

**Treat it.** The two best antifungal creams are Lamisil AT for your feet and Lotrimin AF for your crotch. The latter is more expensive than generic clotrimazole, but Dr. Nasir has found it to have better results. He also suggests Fungoid Tincture. It contains miconazole nitrate, which kills the fungus, and isopropyl alcohol as a drying agent. Just don't quit using it when the itch stops; apply it for another 2 weeks after the last visible sign. "There is a microscopic problem there that must be treated," he says.

A dirty trick: Fungus will sometimes hide under your toenails. If that happens, dribble some regular-flavor Listerine under each nail. "The potency is less than that of the tincture, but it works the same way and is certainly a great home remedy," says Dr. Nasir.

**Prevent it.** Remember, fungi are everywhere, not just on shower tile but also in carpet. Wear sandals in any gym locker room and at poolside: Rough surfaces can cause tiny skin breaks that let the fungi grab hold. (Teva sells several models of antifungal sandals, such as the all-terrain Guide '06 L/C, which contains a permanent zinc treatment to fight bacteria and fungi; about $95, www.teva.com.) And since, like most plant life, fungi thrive where it's wet, try showering at night so your feet are desert dry when you pull on your socks in the morning. Speaking of socks and other similar sweat collectors, consider entering this century by making the switch to breathable, wicking fabrics.

## PRURITUS ANI

We didn't want to say it out loud: This means itchy butt. And it's more common than you might imagine. "I think it's underreported because people are uncomfortable discussing it," says Scott Moses, MD, a family-practice physician in Minnesota who is something of a pruritus ani expert. But it's not the result of wiping like a 5-year-old—just the opposite. It's commonly caused by excessive wiping, which removes protective natural oils, leading to inflammation. "This inflammation is what causes the itching sensation," says Dr. Moses.

**Treat it.** Yep, there's something just for this: Proctofoam HC, a prescription hydrocortisone in aerosol form, which helps ease the inflammation. It involves an applicator tip. (Ask your doctor about it, because we're not going into it here.) Use it after every bowel movement, but for no more than 2 weeks.

**Prevent it.** Use damp toilet paper (you might need something thick like Charmin Ultra or Charmin Aloe & E) or baby wipes (try Cottonelle premoistened flushable wipes). And blot, don't wipe.

## ITCHY SCALP

You have either dry skin or a buildup of yeast called *Pityrosporum* irritating the itch nerves. *Pityrosporum* is always on your skin and loves to feed on dead scalp cells, a.k.a. dandruff.

**Treat it.** Start using a dandruff shampoo containing yeast-killing ketoconazole, such as Nizoral AD antidandruff shampoo. Hair-gel users should go without to see if the gel is what's causing the problem. If it is, use the goop less often, dilute it with water, or look for an allergen-free brand like Vidal Sassoon Contour Gel. And read the labels on shampoo bottles to avoid additives like sodium sulfate and sodium lauryl sulfate, which can strip your scalp of natural oils.

**Prevent it.** The directions for some dandruff shampoos suggest leaving the suds on your scalp for 5 minutes. Dr. Nasir says it's better to lather up once to remove any buildup of dead skin, then rinse and repeat so the shampoo can kill the excess yeast.

## BURNS AND SCABS

As burns and other skin injuries heal, "remodeling" occurs: Dead tissue breaks down and makes space for healthy tissue, and nerves and blood vessels grow along with this new tissue, says Alan Fleischer, MD, chair of dermatology at the Wake Forest University School of Medicine. Once the hard scar tissue forms, nerves are trapped and may be tickled when the tissue stretches or bends, he says. Moreover, the fibroblast cells that make up scar tissue can release chemicals that trigger itch nerves.

**Treat it.** This itching is a sign of healing, so feel encouraged. But if the power of positive thinking doesn't do the job, try Sarna Anti-Itch, an over-the-counter lotion that contains camphor and menthol to help numb the surface of the irritated area. Or you can try Lanacane, which contains another anesthetic, benzocaine—but use it sparingly.

# MEN'S HEALTH QUIZ

## How's Your Mental Toughness?

Take our test to see if your willpower is out to lunch

**1. You blow a layup or flub a toast. Your next move?**
   A. Crack a self-deprecating joke
   B. Punt the ball or unleash obscenities
   C. Shrug and keep going

Composure after a mistake is an important measure of mental toughness says Patrick Cohn, PhD, a "mental game" coach for Peak Performance Sports in Orlando. "If you have an expectation and your performance doesn't match it, you'll become frustrated." The resulting anxiety will weaken your mental game, on and off the court. "You have to let go of expectations," Dr. Cohn says. And when something goes wrong, don't dwell on it.

**2. Which movie hero do you identify with?**
   A. I'm chill, like Clint Eastwood in *Dirty Harry*.
   B. I'm a fighter, like Sylvester Stallone in *Rocky*.
   C. I'm high-strung, like Al Pacino in *Scarface*.

The most relaxed guys are the toughest, says Bill Kipp, a former marine and the owner of FAST Defense, a company that trains people to handle crises. "The mentally tough can respond to any situation spontaneously," he says, "so they stay relaxed during downtime rather than stressing." Meditating for 20 minutes daily clears and sharpens your mind. That's right, marines meditate. Got a problem?

**3. You make eye contact with a beautiful woman at a bar. You . . .**
   A. Smile, but let her come to you
   B. Look away immediately
   C. Approach her with a drink

Confidence is crucial for mental toughness, so build it by overcoming challenges, says Dr. Cohn. "Ask yourself what you've done in the past that proves you can do something today." Take on as many new challenges as possible, whether you're rock climbing, cooking Thai, or turning eye contact into something more.

### 4. You've just been laid off. What's your first move?
A. Sulk, unplug the phone, and pull the shades
B. Invite your pals over; let them cheer you up
C. Trash-talk your boss on your blog

The weak respond to setbacks by hiding or lashing out. "Someone who's mentally tough has the maturity to reach out and ask for help when he needs it," says Kipp. Build a group of strong male friends you can count on. When you're doubting your worth, they'll remind you of the real bottom line.

### Scoring

| | | | |
|---|---|---|---|
| 1. | A= 2 | B=1 | C=3 |
| 2. | A= 3 | B=2 | C=1 |
| 3. | A= 2 | B=1 | C=3 |
| 4. | A= 2 | B=3 | C=1 |

**4–6:** You have a serious case of mental mush.

**7–9:** You're halfway to hard-headed. Suck it up.

**10–12:** You have an iron will. Wield it wisely.

# BURNING QUESTIONS

**Do I need to replace my toothbrush after I've been sick?**

That's the smart play. The flu, the common cold, and strep all can incubate on your toothbrush, prolonging or spreading illness, says Barbara Rich, DDS, FAGD, a spokeswoman for the Academy of General Dentistry. You could play it cheap and still stay healthy, however. Rinse the old brush thoroughly in an antiseptic mouthwash like Listerine, shake off the excess, and let the bristles dry completely. "In warm, moist conditions, the bacteria continue to thrive," says Dr. Rich. And don't overlook your toothpaste. By running your germ-encrusted brush across the toothpaste tube and passing said tube to your girlfriend, you could be passing her the flu as well. Maybe you're cool with that. If not, buy a separate tube for each of you.

**How can I know if I'm a hypochondriac?**

It's not whether you worry about your health; it's how you react when a doctor tells you you're healthy, says *Men's Health* mental-health advisor William Pollack, PhD. If you feel relieved to be disease-free, you are not a hypochondriac. True hypochondriacs stay worried. They have an unshakable, unreasonable belief that they're ill.

**Which fish has the highest omega-3 count?**

Pacific herring tops the omega-3 fish standings with 2 grams per 3-ounce serving. But it's often pickled or smoked, so second-place salmon (1.8 grams) may be a better choice. Sablefish (1.7 grams), sardines (1.2 grams), and mackerel (1.1 grams) round out the most heart-healthy school of fish.

**What needs disinfecting and what's just media hype?**

Germs are everywhere, but only a few make us sick, and they're the ones likely hanging out in kitchens and bathrooms. Sinks are the frat houses of bacterial life: Their moist conditions and constant contact with dirty hands

**NUMBER OF BONES AMERICAN MEN BREAK EACH YEAR: 3 million**

keep them teeming with germs. Disinfect them once a week with half a cup of bleach or a cleaner labeled as a disinfectant and pay special attention to the faucet and handles. In public restrooms, avoid the sink altogether and stick with a hand sanitizer, says Charles Gerba, PhD, professor of environmental microbiology at the University of Arizona.

Phones are another hot spot; they're prime resting locations for airborne, transferable viruses like the common cold. High-contact surfaces, such as shopping-cart handles, pose a chance of picking up a nasty bug; if you're prone to illness, use those wipes that grocery stores provide. Still, you've made it this far without them, so the choice is up to you.

### What is sciatica, and why do I keep getting it?

Sciatica is the term given to pain that radiates down either leg from the base of your spine, often as a result of some kind of damage to the sciatic nerve, which follows the same route. "The most common causes are a narrowing of the spinal column, arthritis, or a pinching of the nerve from a herniated disk or a muscle in your buttocks," says Loren M. Fishman, MD, physiatrist and author of *Relief Is in the Stretch: End Back Pain through Yoga*. "But there's no way to tell for sure without a proper diagnosis." Depending on the root cause, treatment can range from physical therapy and mild medication to epidural steroid injections and even surgery. Exercise, correct lifting technique, and an office chair with good lumbar support are all obvious things that will help you avoid sciatica. Also, take that bulging wallet out of your back pocket. It can cause pressure on the nerve.

### Is coffee causing my acid reflux? I have 3 cups a day.

There's only one way to know for sure: Stop drinking it. "If everything clears up, caffeine was the culprit," says Steven Peikin, MD, head of gastroenterology at Cooper University Hospital in New Jersey. The problem is that coffee (and the caffeine contained therein) is but one of many foods that can trigger acid reflux—others include peppermint, chocolate, nuts, and greasy anything, and it can take up to 30 minutes for the symptoms (heartburn, chest pain, trouble swallowing) to set in. But if you can't do without your cups o' joe, chase them with a stick of gum. A recent study found that chewing gum stimulates enough saliva to neutralize stomach acid that would otherwise flow into the esophagus and cause acid reflux.

### My stomach always gurgles. What's up?

It doesn't mean you're hungry, says *Men's Health* gastroenterology advisor Mark Welton, MD. The rumbling could be caused by incomplete digestion, which leads to excess gas. If it bothers you, try to determine which foods cause the gurgling. Eliminate one food per day—jot down what you eat—to determine the culprit.

## Bottom-line it once and for all: Is cheese bad for me?

No. Cheese gets a bad rap because some varieties contain a potentially lethal trio of saturated fat, sodium, and cholesterol, a combination that can clog your arteries and elevate blood pressure. If you consume it in moderation, however, cheese is healthful. It's a good source of protein, calcium, phosphorus, vitamin D, vitamin A, riboflavin, and vitamin $B_{12}$. Choose string cheese and part-skim mozzarella and ricotta (all low in fat) and reduced-fat hard cheeses, suggests Lisa Tartamella-Kimmel, MS, RD, outpatient nutrition coordinator at Yale–New Haven Hospital.

## What's new in kidney-stone treatment?

The latest procedures are less invasive than traditional surgery, says *Men's Health* urology advisor Larry Lipshultz, MD. State-of-the-art miniature scopes and lasers allow surgeons to extract a stone through the urinary tract without making an incision. Stone-dissolving drugs are also in development.

# FIVE

# CHEAT DEATH

# READ UP ON IT

## The Time Bomb Inside of You

Arm yourself to defuse the explosive that's ticking in your prostate

**by Hamilton Cain**

"He's in the hospital."

"The cancer has spread."

"We're hoping for the best."

It's amazing, the life-changing capacity of a single phone call. Just a minute before, my wife and I were happily packing for a vacation, our tangle of clothes in the middle of the room, the price tag still attached to her new swimsuit. Then came the call from Ellen's mom. Her dad's prostate cancer was back, and it had spread to his spine. We hastily changed our travel plans. Destination: Los Angeles.

A dashing, fit, silver-haired professor of psychology at UCLA, Michael Goldstein had had a brush with prostate cancer 3 years earlier. Although he hadn't suffered the symptoms that sometimes emerge—an unrelenting urge to urinate, a burning sensation when he did—a blood test at his annual physical indicated high levels of prostate-specific antigen, or PSA. His family had been surprised, given the trademark high energy that allowed him to teach graduate seminars, conduct his own research, and fly to and from Europe several times a year to lecture in Rome, London, and Amsterdam. After he opted to have the cancerous gland removed, his doctors pronounced him cured, and he threw himself back, with gusto, into his work, his family, his life.

We arrived in Los Angeles the morning after the phone call and drove straight to the hospital. When we walked into my father-in-law's room, he seemed tired, a trifle sallow, but otherwise still his optimistic, glass-half-full self. A nurse was teaching him to walk with a back brace that looked about as comfortable as a corset. Outside, a dry wind rattled the eucalyptus fronds, but here the air smelled of disinfectants and the light was eternal fluorescent.

I'd last seen him at our wedding, 6 months earlier, on a snowy, breezy afternoon in Manhattan. Ellen walked down the aisle on her father's arm as he radiated paternal pride. At the reception, he charmed the guests with a toast only a father could give: "As a girl, Ellen loved to hear stories, and I always knew she'd marry a man who would regale her with story after story...."

Now, as we tried to summon comforting, cliché-free words, he teetered down the corridor, tracing his right hand along the rail for support. I helped him practice his new steps, his arm slung across my shoulder. A week later, tests confirmed that the cancer had, in fact, spread. Somehow he maintained his confident, cheerful facade, yet the creases around his eyes hinted that he knew. He was, after all, a man of science. The little lifts of good news—We've confined the cancer to just a few spots on the spinal column, some mild radiation will take care of it, the worst thing will be the damned brace—were only temporary lulls in a gathering storm.

In less than 7 months, he was gone.

About 635 men a day are diagnosed with prostate cancer. It's a frightening figure. But perhaps not scary enough, since many young men still dismiss the disease as just another unavoidable side effect of aging.

Here's why you should take it more seriously: Groundbreaking autopsy studies from Wayne State University show that prostate-cancer risk rises 10 percentage points with each passing decade. Thirty-year-olds have a 30 percent chance of carrying a trace of the cancer, forty-somethings a 40 percent chance, and so on. Sure, it usually progresses so slowly that most men die of something else first, but prostate cancer does kill more than 30,000 men annually—1 percent are under the age of 55, and 8 percent are under age 65. More virulent forms, like my father-in-law's, can kill in less than a year.

The prostate gland, scarcely larger than a cherry tomato, is tucked between the bladder and the urethra, ideally situated to perform its primary function: to secrete seminal fluid for ejaculation, so that sperm can be propelled through the urethra and out to begin their mad dash to meet a lonely ovum. It's ironic, then, that a gland that plays such a central role in creating life—greasing the skids, as it were—threatens to end a man's life as well.

The most important men in my life have been dancing around this killer for a few years now. Not only did the disease take my father-in-law at the age of 67, but my own 76-year-old father is at increased risk. His most recent blood test revealed a moderately elevated PSA. My grandfather also developed prostate cancer as he struggled with his final, fatal pneumonia. (He was 92 at the time, so a urologist might say he "lived long enough" to contract the illness.) And, of course, I have the number one risk factor: I'm a man.

My brother-in-law, Peter, knows the danger well, the disease having cut short the lives of two men in his family. Recently, he confided his anxiety: "Dude, I'm toast."

So, on a warm June morning, I visit Daniel Petrylak, MD, an oncologist at Columbia Presbyterian Hospital's Irving Cancer Center in New York City. Dr. Petrylak, a leading prostate-cancer researcher, has helped shape the course of treatment. With me is a list of questions you'd expect a journalist writing a story about prostate cancer to be carrying. But I also carry a second list, one that probably reads a lot like yours:

1. Exactly how at risk am I?
2. Should I have a PSA test?
3. What can I do to reduce my risk?

And then I have a final, more personal question: Could my father-in-law have been saved?

"So you're concerned that you're at risk?" asks Dr. Petrylak, a handsome, dapper man with deep brown eyes. His gaze flits back and forth from me to his computer screen.

"It's been on my mind," I respond.

"How old are you?"

"Just turned 40."

"All men over 50 should have a PSA test," says Dr. Petrylak. "But the earlier a man and his doctor can catch prostate cancer, the broader the range of treatment options."

PSA, a protein manufactured in the prostate, is measured with a simple blood test. Men with prostate cancer, or even enlargement of the prostate, have higher levels of PSA because it rises in response to any type of trauma. Dr. Petrylak explains that a PSA count above 4.0 (as measured in nanograms per milliliter) raises a red flag, although a recent study suggests that a bigger threat is a PSA that rises quickly. (See "Solving the PSA Puzzle," on page 156.)

If the PSA score looks alarmingly elevated, the urologist will usually suggest a biopsy of the gland. Likewise if he detects a suspicious lesion during a

(continued on page 152)

# WHAT'S YOUR RISK?

You're looking at the best self-test for prostate cancer, short of a DIY digital rectal exam. Formulated by the Prostate Cancer Research Foundation of Canada, it analyzes all the relevant risk factors (and reducers), then spits out a score. When we polled our urology advisors, they agreed: It can ID a prostate in peril.

**1.** How old are you?
   A. Under age 40 (–5 points)
   B. 40–49 (0 points)
   C. 50–59 (+6 points)
   D. 60–70 (+8 points)
   E. Over 70 (+10 points)

**2.** What's your body-mass index (BMI)? Calculate your BMI at www.menshealth.com/BMI.
   A. 24.9 or lower (0 points)
   B. 25–29.9 (+3 points)
   C. Higher than 29.9 (+6 points)

**3.** What's your ethnicity?
   A. Asian/Pacific Islander (0 points)
   B. White non-Latino (+5 points)
   C. White Latino (+3 points)
   D. Black (+8 points)
   E. Other (0 points)

**4.** Where did you spend most of your life until age 21?
   A. North America (+8 points)
   B. Northern Europe (Scandinavia) or Western Europe (+8 points)
   C. Southern or Eastern Europe (+2 points)
   D. Asia/Pacific Islands (–5 points)
   E. Other (0 points)

**5.** Has your father or a brother been diagnosed with prostate cancer?
   A. No (0 points)
   B. Father (+6 points)
   C. Brother (+8 points)
   D. Father and brother (+12 points)
If you answered "A" to question 5, skip to question 7.

**6.** How old was the family member who was diagnosed youngest?
   A. Age 49 or younger (+8 points)
   B. 50–59 (+6 points)
   C. 60–69 (+3 points)
   D. 70 or older (0 points)

**7.** Do you regularly take nonsteroidal anti-inflammatory drugs, such as aspirin or ibuprofen?

    A. Yes (–1 point)

    B. No (0 points)

**8.** How often do you exercise? (Twenty minutes of weight lifting or cardio work equals 1 session.)

    A. 1–3 sessions per week (+2 points)

    B. 4–6 sessions per week (0 points)

    C. 7 or more sessions per week (–2 points)

**9.** How often do you eat foods high in saturated fats, such as fatty red or processed meats?

    A. Once a week or less (0 points)

    B. 2–3 times a week (+1 point)

    C. 4–5 times a week (+3 points)

    D. 6–10 times a week (+5 points)

**10.** How often do you eat foods loaded with lycopene (grapefruit, mango, papaya, watermelon, and tomato products)?

    A. Once a week or less (0 points)

    B. 2–3 times a week (–1 point)

    C. 4–5 times a week (–2 points)

    D. 6–10 times a week (–3 points)

**11.** How often do you eat foods rich in cancer-fighting phytochemicals (soy products, broccoli, and brussels sprouts)?

    A. Once a week or less (0 points)

    B. 2–3 times a week (–1 point)

    C. 4–5 times a week (–2 points)

    D. 6–10 times a week (–3 points)

**12.** How often do you eat foods rich in omega-3 fatty acids (tuna, salmon, sardines, walnuts, and flaxseed)?

    A. Once a week or less (0 points)

    B. 2–3 times a week (–1 point)

    C. 4–5 times a week (–2 points)

    D. 6–10 times a week (–3 points)

**13.** Does your diet include foods high in zinc (whole grains, poultry, fish, soy, lentils, and beans)?

    A. Yes (–1 point)

    B. No (0 points)

**14.** Does your diet include foods high in selenium (mushrooms, cod, shrimp, and tuna)?

    A. Yes (–3 points)

    B. No (0 points)

*(continued)*

# WHAT'S YOUR RISK? (CONT.)

**15.** Does your diet include calcium-rich foods (milk, cheese, and yogurt)?
    A. Yes (+2 points)
    B. No (0 points)

**16.** Does your diet include foods high in vitamin D (fish oils, shrimp)?
    A. Yes (–1 point)
    B. No (0 points)

**17.** Does your diet include foods high in vitamin E (peanut butter, almonds, sunflower seeds)?
    A. Yes (–2 points)
    B. No (0 points)

**18.** Have you ever worked in an industry in which you might have been exposed to pesticides, herbicides, PCBs, lead, or asbestos?
    A. Yes (+1 point)
    B. No (0 points)

## Scoring

**0–10 points:** Low risk

The odds of cancer infiltrating your well-guarded gland are enviably low. Just don't become complacent and drop your defenses; this disease will wait a lifetime for an opening.

**11–20 points:** Low to moderate risk

Sure, Vegas would pick you over prostate cancer, but there's room for an upset. Review your answers, paying attention to where you scored high in factors you can control. Make it your mission to improve your score in two of these areas.

**21–34 points:** Moderate to high risk

If this were a Homeland Security alert, the threat of sleeper cells would put your prostate at Code Orange. You need to act. In addition to losing weight and adding exercise, commit to hitting negative numbers (or zero) in every diet category.

**35 or more points:** High risk

Your prostate is a cancer magnet. If you're age 40 or older, you should be having annual digital rectal exams and PSA tests. Haven't gotten around to it? What on your to-do list is more important than "Save my life"? If you're younger than 40, talk to a urologist about a baseline PSA test. And whatever your age, start slashing your score.

digital rectal exam. After the biopsy, the tissue is analyzed under a microscope. If it's found to be cancerous, the clinicians assign a Gleason score, which ranges from 2 to 10 and indicates the kind of cancer that's present and whether it could aggressively spread to other parts of the body. This grading system, developed by pathologist Donald Gleason, MD, in 1977, is used with a system of stages (from 1 to 4) to steer a man to a preferred form of treatment. Depending on the cancer's severity, a patient can choose from various options, such as a radical prostatectomy (surgical removal of the gland), radiation therapy (nuking the cancer), surgical castration (removal of the testicles to halt the production of testosterone, which can fuel the cancer), hormone therapy (sometimes called chemical castration), or a combination of these treatments.

When confronted with a PSA count of 7.0, my father-in-law opted for a prostatectomy. Soon after, his PSA level dropped back to near zero, and his doctor declared that the disease had been beaten. For weeks, my father-in-law joked that he'd avoided the ultimate male fear, "the snip-snip." He pushed ahead with his active life, traveling from Los Angeles to New York City to see Ellen and me, and then on to Europe, where he lectured on schizophrenia and bipolar disorder—and found a way to fly in and out of Brussels, where his son lived, in order to dandle his new granddaughter on his knee.

What he didn't know was that his prostate cancer wasn't beaten. It was hiding.

"We now think of cancer as a genetic disease."

That's William Isaacs, MD, a leading prostate-cancer researcher at Johns Hopkins University. According to Dr. Isaacs, 91 percent of all prostate cancers are sparked by DNA that becomes corroded over the course of a man's life (more on that in a moment). The other 9 percent are also triggered by a hiccup in the helix, except that this flaw is passed down from generation to generation. In fact, if a man younger than 55 develops prostate cancer, there's a good chance that he has his dad to thank. More than 40 percent of those cases, researchers now believe, involve one of several mutant genes passed from fathers to sons.

Here's another way to look at Dr. Isaacs's breakdown: Nine in 10 men who develop prostate cancer were actually born with healthy genetic blueprints for their prostates. In these men, DNA damage results from what Dr. Isaacs calls "somatic changes triggered by environmental issues." In other words, diet, smoking, lack of exercise—all the gremlins *Men's Health* magazine continually warns you about.

Another of these "environmental issues," and potentially the most powerful of all, is infection. "Our natural immunities kill bacteria effectively—without them, we couldn't live," explains Dr. Isaacs. "But our immune responses are also potent in altering our own DNA over a lifetime. Call it 'collateral damage.'" So, in an effort to completely wipe out one enemy, our bodies may inadvertently set the stage for another, more powerful opponent to rise from the glandular rubble.

The emerging hypothesis—researchers shy away from the word *consensus*—is that the presence and virulence of prostate cancer are intertwined with inflammation, the cellular signpost that indicates an immune reaction. And, oddly, the best tool for measuring prostate inflammation may be a heart test.

For several years now, smart cardiologists have been assessing their patients' blood levels of C-reactive protein (CRP), one of the body's main inflammation markers. High levels—over 3 milligrams per liter—are generally considered to be a risk factor for a heart attack, since inflammation can signal the presence of arterial plaque. So doctors at Mount Sinai Medical Center in New York City theorized that if elevated CRP levels could predict heart trouble, then they might also help forecast prostate cancer. The docs were right: After analyzing the blood work of 114 men with prostate cancer, the researchers discovered that the men's CRP and PSA scores rose and fell in unison.

More research is needed to confirm this connection, but the implications are significant. Not only might CRP testing be used as a tool for diagnosing prostate cancer, but it could also serve as an early warning system that helps men avoid the disease.

Just as intriguing, says Dr. Isaacs, is how an out-of-whack immune response may figure into the inherited form of the disease. He had been studying families rife with prostate cancer for years when, in 2002, he and his colleagues made a discovery on chromosome 1. Through their analysis of about 200 families, they identified RNASEL, a gene that encodes an enzyme

## A KILLER'S HIT LIST

When prostate cancer spreads, these are its top targets

**Liver:** In one in four patients with advanced cancer, malignant prostate cells can spread to the liver and, in the worst cases, cause fatal liver failure.

**Hip bones:** Cancer cells that lodge in the pelvis, spine, or other parts of the skeleton release substances that eat away at bone, making it brittle and causing pain.

**Lymph nodes:** Invasion of nearby nodes means the cancer now has the means to spread to distant sites via the network of vessels and nodes that collects excess fluid, or lymph, from all parts of the body.

**Bladder:** The first stop for cancer that has escaped the prostate is often right next door: the semen-storing seminal vesicles at either side of the gland, or the neck of the bladder.

**PERCENTAGE CHANCE A 30-YEAR-OLD HAS OF HAVING PROSTATE CANCER: 30**

whose job it is to prevent viral infection. A mutation in the gene basically opens up a "pathway" to prostate inflammation.

Still, Dr. Isaacs believes that, unlike with BRCA1, the gene whose mutated form almost always accurately predicts breast cancer, there's no one genetic flaw that causes prostate cancer. "Prostate cancer may be more complex than breast cancer," he says. "We know that many genes are affected."

I wonder aloud whether RNASEL or some other obscure genetic culprit caused my father-in-law's death—after all, his own father suffered from the disease for years before succumbing in the '80s. When I mention my father-in-law's case, Dr. Isaacs perks up. Apparently, even when you take DNA into account, it's uncommon for a healthy, active man in his mid-sixties to fall under the scythe of the disease in a matter of months. "Guys like your father-in-law...these guys fascinate us," he says. "Clinically speaking, we really can't explain them. The example I always use is Frank Zappa, who was diagnosed at 52 and went quickly."

I smile grimly to myself as Dr. Isaacs links these rare cases. He's conjured a couple of fond adolescent memories: the famous Zappa album cover *Ship Arriving Too Late to Save a Drowning Witch*; the annoyingly catchy lyrics of "Valley Girl" blaring ubiquitously from Trans Am stereos in the summer of 1982; barf out; gag me with a spoon. Frank Zappa had lived in the Hollywood Hills, where on warm afternoons his children, Moon Unit and Dweezil, tagged along with other neighborhood kids, roaming the box canyons high above a blanket of smog. I now wonder if they remember one of their playmates, a slender, angular girl with parted Marcia Brady hair and a quick, sarcastic wit.

The girl who'd one day become my wife.

For a man weaned on hush puppies and barbecue, I've struggled with being married to a strict vegetarian, grumbling at the menu restrictions she's cruelly imposed on me, such as steamed spinach and stir-fried tofu. In the long run, though, I may have her to thank for a healthy, cancer-free life.

A colleague of Dr. Isaacs's, Bill Nelson, MD, has researched the role of diet in prostate cancer and offers a few rules to, in the fullest sense of the

## SOLVING THE PSA PUZZLE

### How doctors may be misreading your most important blood marker

Measuring PSA is simple: Draw blood, send to lab. What's complicated is interpreting the results.

In 2005, a study of 1,308 men published in the *Journal of the National Cancer Institute* showed that even men with PSAs greater than 10.0 nanograms per milliliter (ng/ml)—well above the 4.0 ng/ml danger threshold used by urologists—were biopsied for cancer that wasn't there. This has led some doctors, such as Gilbert Welch, MD, MPH, the lead study author, to argue for raising the PSA cutoff point.

Other scientists disagree. They point to a 2004 study published in the *New England Journal of Medicine* that found evidence of cancer in 15 percent of men with PSAs below 4.0 ng/ml. In this case, the magic number for disease detection would be 2.5.

So where does this leave us? "No one should use a single PSA result to trigger a biopsy," says Anthony D'Amico, MD, lead author of a study showing that how fast PSA levels rise from an initial result of 4.0 ng/ml or higher may be a bigger clue to cancer. "If it goes up by as much as 2.0 ng/ml 3 months later, a biopsy is in order," says Dr. D'Amico. And if you're a younger guy, he recommends a PSA test once at age 35, so that you already have a baseline measurement.

word, live by. First, given that the common denominator for the disease seems to be inflammation and the body's autoimmune responses, he pounds the pulpit for foods whose chemistry can combat infection: fruits and vegetables—the "broccoli as cure for cancer" idea in vogue for the past decade. Noting that Southeast Asian men have much lower rates of prostate cancer—and that their first- and second-generation immigrant sons in Western countries have rates comparable to those of native-born Caucasians—he also preaches the Gospel of Soy.

"And think about taking supplements, like selenium and vitamin E, as well as such anti-inflammatory medications as aspirin and ibuprofen," he says. And, for God's sake, he notes, please avoid charbroiled meat; carcinogens in it have been shown to disproportionately cause prostate cancer in lab studies.

Another way to reduce the risk is to engage the prostate's self-cleaning cycle. Researchers in Australia recently queried more than 1,000 men with prostate cancer about their ejaculation rates and compared the results with data obtained from a comparable group of healthy men. These researchers discovered that men who ejaculated frequently between the ages of 20 and 50 were at markedly lower risk of developing prostate cancer. Even more provocatively, men in their 20s who ejaculated at least five times a week were one-third less likely to develop aggressive prostate cancer during their mature years. All those high-school PE-class jokes assume new meaning when I ponder the clear health benefits of chronic masturbation.

Conclusion: Prostate cancer often can be prevented through the basics of a healthy diet and vigorous exercise, whether one plays on an intramural basketball team or in the privacy of the bathroom with the skilled assistance of the December Playmate of the Month.

And if prevention fails? Detection can succeed in saving us.

"The incidence in younger men is soaring," observes Dr. Isaacs, "but only because detection methods have improved exponentially." However, he adds, this also raises new questions. "How do we use screening effectively? Are we overdiagnosing and overtreating, especially in younger patients? There are so many controversial areas of prostate cancer."

Like other clinicians, Dr. Petrylak feels the PSA test has its limits in predicting the presence of cancer: "We need better, more specific tests at this point." He frequently consults with David Bostwick, whose eponymous Bostwick Laboratories has identified a new marker in urine and has brought the first non-PSA test onto the market.

Created in the Netherlands by Jack Schalken, MD, the uPM3 test—"the first real prostate test to come out of the genomics revolution"—requires massaging of the prostate gland through a digital rectal examination. This dislodges cells and bits of tissue, which are then flushed out into the urine. The patient immediately heads off to the bathroom to pee into a special cup, where the expressed cells and tissues are collected. The urine specimen is then ferried to a lab, where clinicians must analyze the cell's RNA within 72 hours—a more complicated and time-consuming process than looking at PSA but also more likely to yield an accurate diagnosis.

Dr. Bostwick says it's an exciting time for early detection. "Molecular biology is revolutionizing medicine. In prostate cancer, the molecular era began with PSA and has progressed to PCA3Plus, which tests men's urine for mRNA specific for prostate cancer. It has a high positive predictive value (if it is positive, a man has a 57 percent chance of having prostate cancer) and a high negative predictive value (if it is negative, a man has an 83 percent chance of not having prostate cancer). It is the next-generation screening test for prostate cancer."

In my father-in-law's case, the usual tools for detecting prostate cancer

(continued on page 160)

# THE TUMOR TAMERS
## Your array of options when the diagnosis is cancer

### Radical prostatectomy

After slicing you from belly button to pubic bone, the surgeon removes your prostate and any diseased tissue around it. New laparoscopic techniques—with or without a hand from robotic arms—result in smaller cuts, minimizing recovery time.

**How effective is it?** Among 2,091 men with tumors confined to the prostate, 72 percent stayed cancer-free for 10 years, according to a Johns Hopkins analysis. Laparoscopic techniques seem comparable.

**Any problems?** Studies of patients in the mid-1990s found that 5 years later, roughly 80 percent had erectile problems, and 15 percent had leaky bladders. Today, new techniques can reduce those rates.

**Whom is it best for?** Men in whom the tumor takes up at least 5 percent of the prostate but hasn't spread beyond it. When compared with radiation therapy alone, it gives men whose cancer has advanced slightly past the gland's perimeter a 79 percent chance of surviving an extra 10 years.

### Chemotherapy

Chemical warfare for cancer. This is any oral or intravenous drug that combats the disease. The most promising agent right now is the breast-cancer drug Taxotere (docetaxel), which stops malignant cells from multiplying.

**How effective is it?** In studies published last year in the *New England Journal of Medicine*, men with hormone-resistant prostate cancer who were put on Taxotere-based regimens survived about 19 months, 2 to 3 months longer than men on chemo treatments that included mitoxantrone.

**Any problems?** Nausea and vomiting, hair loss, diarrhea, mouth sores, and fatigue.

**Whom is it best for?** Men whose spreading cancer doesn't respond to radiation and is resistant to androgen deprivation.

### Radiation therapy

Call it the nuclear option. High-energy x-rays from either tightly focused beams or radioactive seeds are used to kill cancer cells.

**How effective is it?** Men younger than 60 treated with external-beam radiotherapy (EBRT) had a 7-year cancer-free survival rate near 80 percent, say researchers at Memorial Sloan-Kettering Cancer Center. Younger men treated with radioactive seeds had a better than 90 percent chance of staying cancer-free after 7 years, according to a separate study.

**Any problems?** It's estimated that half of men become impotent 5 years after EBRT. A study in the *International Journal of Radiation Oncology* found that 1 year after seeding, 60 percent of men report bladder-control problems, and 80 percent experience impotence.

**Whom is it best for?** Men with gland-confined cancer that's at low risk of spreading who don't want or can't have surgery. The drawback to radiation is that it takes years to know for certain if the cancer is still active.

## Cryosurgery

Guided by ultrasound, doctors slide several hollow probes into the gland, then pump in ultracold (below −40°F) liquid. The prostate is then thawed, refrozen, and thawed again.

**How effective is it?** This generation of cryo is still new, but a study of 590 Michigan hospital patients with organ-confined or locally advanced cancer put their odds of remaining cancer-free at between 60 and 70 percent after 7 years.

**Any problems?** "You have to freeze the area slightly outside the prostate to get rid of any cancer in the margins," says Judd Moul, MD, chief of urologic surgery at Duke University Medical Center. "That can damage the nerves that control erections." Freezing may also create a hole between the rectum and the bladder, which can cause urine leaks.

**Whom is it best for?** Men whose prostate cancer has returned following radiation therapy. "You can freeze a prostate even after it's been irradiated," says Dr. Moul.

## Androgen deprivation

A euphemism for the C word—*castration*—either with drugs or, in very advanced cases, surgery. The goal is to suppress the supply of testosterone and other androgen-based hormones that can fuel prostate cancer.

**How effective is it?** Studies suggest that androgen deprivation combined with external radiation treatment can improve survival in men whose cancer either is likely to spread just outside the gland or already has. It can also ease bone pain and urinary obstructions.

**Any problems?** Hot flashes, breast growth, shrinking muscle mass, fatigue, depression, weight gain, and decreased HDL cholesterol.

**Whom is it best for?** Men with cancer that's likely to spread and who are receiving radiation, and men with advanced cancer who suffer from bone pain. "Hormone therapy usually doesn't cure, but it keeps the cancer down for a while," says Paul Lange, MD, chairman of urology at the University of Washington School of Medicine.

## Expectant management

The option formerly known as "watchful waiting." In cases in which the cancer is extremely small and slow in growing, your doctor may monitor your condition, waiting to begin treatment until symptoms appear or the cancer progresses.

**How effective is it?** As long as the cancer stays put, you avoid unnecessary treatment and possible side effects.

**Any problems?** You need a digital rectal exam and a PSA measurement every 6 months, and needle biopsies at 6 and 18 months, or more frequently.

**Whom is it best for?** Men with a very small amount of cancer who are in a low-risk category, says Dr. Lange. "If you're in your 40s, I would say no; if you're in your 60s, it can be an option."

failed to uncover his disease. And then, despite the arsenal of weapons available, his urologist was unable to eradicate every last malignant cell. As I discovered, one cell is all it takes.

In a weird twist, the only treatment that might have offered my father-in-law any hope of survival was the same one that's currently saving women by the score: the breast-cancer drug Taxotere (docetaxel). Lab studies in the late 1990s showed that the medication was surprisingly effective at combating late-term prostate cancer, prompting Dr. Petrylak to conduct his own trial. In 2004, he published his results in the *New England Journal of Medicine*, in which he described the clear benefits of a chemotherapy regimen based on Taxotere. After cranking his data through various algorithms, he calculated a 20 percent spike in the survival rate among patients. Just as significant, he detailed dramatic improvements in quality of life, despite such debilitating side effects as osteoporosis and loss of sexual function. Dr. Petrylak acknowledges feeling a bittersweet pang when he hears a common refrain from his patients: "Doc, I feel like someone has taken the wind out of my sails."

He's now concentrating on enhancing the benefits of Taxotere with a second drug. In a new blind trial, he'll develop a regimen for late-term prostate-cancer patients, combining Taxotere with Revlimid (lenalidomide); the latter is akin to thalidomide, the drug originally used in pregnant women in the late 1950s to temper morning sickness but discontinued when many of the babies born to those women had birth defects. Dr. Petrylak hopes that, taken in tandem, Taxotere and Revlimid will reduce the cancer's toxicity and increase the efficacy of the treatment program. He expects the trial to grow to as many as 36 patients.

As much as I want Dr. Petrylak's trial to be a success, what I want even more is to avoid becoming one of its participants. When I mention this to him, he concurs with Dr. Nelson's recommendation: "A heart-healthy diet is a prostate-healthy diet." More important, a man should undergo an annual prostate examination, with semiannual PSA tests, beginning at age 40 if there's a strong family history of prostate cancer.

In the fall of 2004—calmly, uneventfully, with no abrupt outbreak of gray hair around the temples, no crow's-feet around the eyes—I passed the milestone of my 40th birthday. One evening some weeks later, my wife and I sat down on the couch after dinner, and while she watched over my shoulder, I jotted down a list on a notepad: blood pressure, cholesterol, colonoscopy, prostate exam. The following afternoon, I was heading into Manhattan for my yearly physical, and I'd made a solemn promise to my wife.

Ellen pushed a wing of hair out of her eyes. "You make sure you check in with Dr. Beautyman about everything."

"I will."

She rapped me on the shoulder. "That means a prostate exam, too."

"Dr. B. will probably refer me to a urologist." I knew that might take a while: the referral back-and-forth, the scheduling of an appointment, the rescheduling of the appointment because one of our newborn twin sons is sick. I had only a vague notion what the exam would entail but was content to put it off ad infinitum. With any luck, I could draw this out until my 41st birthday.

As I sat on the examination table the next afternoon, stripped to my skivvies under the paper gown, my strategy was firm. Dr. Beautyman strode into the room, a tall, fashionable woman in her 50s, a silk skirt and Manolo Blahniks showing from beneath her lab coat. We exchanged small talk as she snaked her stethoscope across my chest and back, listening to my heart and lungs. The kids are all doing well, no real problems this year, weight 155 pounds, blood pressure up a smidgen but normal for a 40-year-old man. She asked me to stand and slip my boxer shorts to the floor, turn my head, and cough while she checked my testicles for a hernia.

As I tugged the shorts back up, relieved that I'd gotten past that awkward moment, I broached the subject. "Now that I'm 40, Dr. Beautyman, do you recommend yearly prostate exams?"

A frown creased her face. "Did your father have prostate cancer?"

"No, but he has had an elevated PSA count. My father-in-law actually died of it, an unusually virulent case."

"I see," she said. She tapped her toe on the linoleum floor while making notes on my chart. I began to peel away the gown and reach toward the examination-room door, where my jeans, shirt, and peacoat hung from a hook.

"Don't get dressed yet," she said. She swiveled on her stool, stood, and placed the chart on top of the credenza. "Hop back onto the table and pull down your shorts, face the wall, and bring your knees to your chest." She rummaged through the credenza's lower drawer.

"I'm sorry?"

"Up on the table," she said. I heard the thwack of a rubber glove.

I lay on my side with my face to the wall, slid my shorts down below my ankles, and with one arm hugged my knees to my chest. The wall was painted beige, that colorless color.

I felt her hand on my hip, steadying my rear end as she eased her fingers in and thrust forward, a doctor's skilled, practiced technique. The shock lifted me an inch off the table's vinyl surface. For an instant, I felt her squeeze deep inside me, palming the soft contours of a ball I'd scarcely been aware I had.

A sharp pang of pain, a star shooting past the edge of sight.

"No suspicious lumps anywhere. You're good to go until next year."

She withdrew and I looked back quickly, saw a bright stain as she stripped off the glove and tossed it into a garbage canister.

"You can get dressed now. I'll call you as soon as I get the blood work back," she said. "If there's anything abnormal, we can discuss it then."

Back home, I sat on the couch, a twin propped in the crook of each arm, their hands flailing about their faces in hunger. There was no residual soreness from the exam, no pain. And no cause for concern. I should be grateful.

But instead, I knew I'd only embarked on a voyage that would last the rest of my life, a quintessentially male experience, one shared by millions of men all over the world. I glanced down into the clear blue stares of my babies. Some day, I knew, they'd join me in the journey.

# Defeating Heart Disease

We've glimpsed the future of heart-disease care, and it is astonishing

**by Christopher McDougall**

I may be the last American man to die of a heart attack. That's not science fiction or fatalism. It's the latest dispatch from medicine's version of the space race, a rapidly accelerating competition of genetic, chemical, and technological innovations that has positioned us, today, within a few years of completely wiping out the number one killer in the Western world.

"There won't be such a thing as a heart attack within the next 10 years," says Eric Topol, MD, chief of cardiology at the Cleveland Clinic, consistently one of the country's top cardiac hospitals. "We're on the verge of making it extinct. We're now at the point where I can say, with confidence, that one of the greatest medical revolutions of the century is about to begin."

Vanquishing an ailment as lethal and inscrutable as heart disease may sound fantastic. But a similar medical miracle has been performed before, and not so long ago. In 1920, the leading cause of death was tuberculosis, which was widely considered incurable. Heard of anyone in the United States dying of "the wasting disease" lately?

But the good news does have a grim exception: One unique type of cardiac sufferer has proven resistant to every new procedure. No one is particularly hopeful of finding a cure for these individuals, either, since every approach so far has failed. Unfortunately, I recently found out I'm a member of this special group. If Dr. Topol's timing is correct, one of us will become a sad medical footnote: the last victim of a killer that can no longer kill.

Here's my profile: I'm 43, I'm in good shape, and I haven't been sick in decades. I haven't had a physical since MTV debuted—25 years, to be exact. I've never had a reason to check my cholesterol, blood pressure, body-mass index, or resting heart rate. My sister and father have some kind of minor arrhythmia, but otherwise, there is no heart disease in my family. At least, not as far as I know; I've never gathered a family medical history.

"You're exactly the guy we worry about—the guy who's dead before we have a chance to save you," says Roger S. Blumenthal, MD, director of preventive cardiology at Johns Hopkins Hospital. "It doesn't matter what wizardry we come up with if you never come through the door till you're cold."

To discover what condition my heart is really in and what kind of lifesaving miracles I might be missing out on, I visited five of the top cardiac centers in the country—Johns Hopkins, Texas Heart Institute, the Cleveland Clinic, Duke University Medical Center, and New York Presbyterian Hospital—and put myself through some of the most advanced cardiac screenings available in the world.

For now, at least, my immersion in all things arterial has removed me from the at-risk group of men who ignore their cardiac health. But it's also turned up some disturbing results I never would have expected.

## FIRST, FIVE FACTS ABOUT THE SILENT KILLER'S M.O.

1. Heart disease isn't just clogged arteries. It's any condition that impedes cardiac bloodflow, so add inflammation, abnormal heart rhythms, a weakened heart muscle, and eroding arteries to the danger list.

2. A heart attack isn't your heart straining to pump enough blood; it's your heart straining to get enough. The heart receives oxygenated blood, like every other organ, but when the arteries that deliver that blood are blocked, the heart quickly suffocates and flatlines.

3. Cholesterol won't kill you. What kills you is a genetic tendency toward fragile arteries that develop cracks in their linings, allowing assorted circulatory gunk to become lodged behind the arterial wall. Eventually, this pile of plaque erupts back into the bloodstream, causing a fatal clot.

4. This year, heart disease will take out nearly a half million American men—more than seven times the total number of U.S. casualties in Vietnam.

5. Despite all the defibrillators now stationed in health-club weight rooms and at basketball courts, one out of every three men who has a heart attack will die from it. You have better odds sticking a bullet in a revolver, spinning the chamber, and playing Russian roulette.

## IF YOUR BLOOD COULD TALK

It's the cardiologist's catch-22: You can't treat a patient's heart disease until it's been diagnosed, but by the time there's something to diagnose—high LDL cholesterol, a lesion in an artery, a blockage—the patient is already in danger. That's why the top priority of heart docs is to find ways to take a sneak peek at the machinery and figure out who's heading toward trouble—before the trouble begins.

"DNA testing isn't quite ready for prime time, but we're close," says Dr. Topol. "Once we identify the genetic strands that indicate arteries with a tendency to crack, your blood can speak up and tell us not only whether you're at risk but also if your kids are, and their kids."

Dr. Topol estimates that it will take less than a decade to decipher the coronary artery's genetic code. But in the meantime, down in the Cleveland Clinic's basement laboratories, one of his colleagues has discovered an entirely different technique for making our blood talk.

When I first meet Stanley Hazen, MD, PhD, with his short, Lou Albano build, I can't help but think that he might want to get out of the lab and invest a little more sweat equity in his own cardiac health. But, then again, if he'd spent the past few years pumping iron instead of probing arteries, he might never have developed the MPO test: a faster, more accurate way to detect heart disease, with the prick of a pin.

As the director of preventive cardiology and rehabilitation for the Cleveland Clinic, Dr. Hazen realized that testing for high cholesterol indicates only the possibility of heart disease, not the probability. So he decided to beam his focus directly on the hot spots: the artery walls. He was looking for a coronary pilot fish—some kind of bodily reaction that shows up before the Big Killer is about to make an appearance. What he discovered is that when a cholesterol-packed artery becomes inflamed, a white-blood-cell enzyme called myeloperoxidase, or MPO, also appears.

"Some 70 percent of heart attacks are caused by inflamed plaque that slightly narrows the vessel, not plaque that builds up to the point of blocking bloodflow," explains Dr. Hazen. "Current tests look for narrowing of the arteries, but that means the damage has already been done." By testing for MPO, he discovered that he could detect unhealthy arteries a lot sooner.

The immediate benefits are enormous: A simple MPO blood test means that emergency-room doctors can quickly and accurately assess every patient who complains of chest pain and determine in minutes whether it's a matter of life or death or a case of acid indigestion. In fact, in September 2005, the first MPO test went on the market for hospital use.

MPO analysis also could be crucial for long-term cardiac risk, Dr. Hazen adds. "Why wait until middle age to start aggressive testing and therapy?" he asks. "We have medicines that have been shown to be safe to use for 30 years. If you wait until the problem presents, the horse is already out of the barn."

## ARTERIAL SHOW-AND-TELL

"After my first look inside a 20-year-old's heart, I never ate ice cream again," says Steven Nissen, MD, a cardiac-imaging specialist at the Cleveland Clinic. "I was horrified at the plaque that's already building up, even when we're young."

Dr. Nissen's wake-up call to the perils of ice-cream consumption came by way of a diagnostic tool that he helped develop: intravascular ultrasound (IVUS), the smallest medical imaging device ever created. This miniature sound probe is snaked inside a patient's arteries, where, like a sonar scanner aimed at the bottom of the sea, it sends out signals and turns the echoes into images. IVUS was first widely used in 1990, but only recently has it been implemented widely enough for comparative data to be compiled. What it offers is a detailed look at every arterial abnormality in its path—plaque, scabbed-over lesions, clotted blood.

Dr. Nissen, whose trim waist testifies to his ice-cream vow and after-hours treadmill miles, first used IVUS to examine the hearts of young accident victims and was shocked by what he found. "Here," he says by way of demonstration, flicking on his desk monitor to show me an interior view of the heart of a 33-year-old man who seemed to be in perfect health before his motorcycle crash. "Take a look at that artery."

He points to something that could be the "before" photo in a Drano ad: a slim pipe whose interior walls are coated so thickly with a milky white paste, it looks half closed. "Everyone thought heart disease was something that came on quickly, but we discovered that plaque starts to accrue almost from birth," he says. "Among people in their twenties, we found that 37 percent already have significant buildup."

IVUS, however, shows only the inside of an artery. For a detailed look at the entire heart, Johns Hopkins Hospital and the Cleveland Clinic recently acquired the world's most powerful computed tomography scanner, otherwise known as a 64-slice CT scanner. Within 10 seconds, it can create a colorized, 3-D computer image of the entire heart by taking 64 x-ray cross-sections and instantly stacking them one on top of the other.

"It's better than an angiogram or intravascular ultrasound because it's noninvasive and allows you to see inside and outside of the arterial wall," says Joao Lima, MD, the director of cardiovascular imaging at Johns Hopkins. "That's why this is a magical time for heart imaging—in the time it takes you to yawn, we can see every corner of your heart."

The 64-slice CT scan is so effective, it solved a near-lethal mystery at the Cleveland Clinic and helped save a staffer's life. "We have a male nurse here, a guy in his early 40s in just super shape, who had chest pains only when he argued with his boss," says Mario Garcia, MD, director of cardiovascular imaging at the Cleveland Clinic. "It never bothered him at home or in the

gym, only when he had to deal with job stress. He went for an electrocardiogram, and it came up clear."

Ordinarily, a case like this would be chalked up to muscle pain, acid
reflux, or joint strain, and the patient would be sent home with Pepto-Bismol
and a pat on the back. This time, Dr. Garcia ran the nurse through the new
64-slice CT scan and discovered a major blockage in one of his coronary arteries. Surgeons were able to open the artery with a stent—a self-expanding
steel-mesh tube—and prevent what would probably have been a surprise
heart attack.

So why doesn't everyone hustle over to Hopkins and get a 64-slice scan,
just in case? Well, there are a few sticking points. One is radiation. "Until we
find a way to lower the radiation exposure, we're limited to giving a patient no

## NATURAL HEART HEALERS

Unlike the space-age treatments discussed here, these natural healers have
stood the test of time.

**Policosanol.** Canadian researchers found that taking 5 to 20 milligrams of this
sugarcane compound daily lowered LDL cholesterol by as much as 31 percent
while raising HDL by up to 29 percent. Consider it if your total cholesterol is
between 200 and 239 milligrams per deciliter, says *Men's Health* advisor John
Elefteriades, MD.

**Niacin.** This B vitamin is an A-list artery cleaner. It raises HDL cholesterol and
lowers triglycerides more than most statins, according to University of Rochester
researchers. And if you combine niacin with a statin, the effect is even more
impressive—15 percent better than with a statin alone. Aim for 500 to 1,500 milligrams daily.

**Peppers.** A Korean study shows that giving rats the human equivalent of 246
milligrams of capsaicin—the heat in hot peppers—lowered their LDL levels by
52 percent. "The effects may be the same in humans," says *Men's Health* advisor
P. K. Shah, MD. Try Nature's Way cayenne pepper supplement.

**Acupuncture.** It might seem counterintuitive, but being stuck with needles
can lower your blood pressure (by as much as 50 percent in lab rats). "The mechanism isn't well understood, but it probably has to do with lowering stress," says
*Men's Health* advisor Eric Topol, MD. *Note:* Do not try this at home; find a certified
acupuncturist at www.acufinder.com.

**Bilberry.** Compared with other berry extracts, bilberry contains twice the
amount of anthocyanins, plant compounds that block the oxidation of LDL cholesterol and prevent inflammation of arteries, says Dr. Shah. Take 480 milligrams of
Nature's Fingerprint bilberry supplement from GNC daily to keep blood vessels
clear and calm.

more than one CT scan a year," says Dr. Lima. He's constantly turning away "the wealthy worried," he says, because if they really needed an x-ray or CT scan in the following few months, the cancer risk would be too great.

The other problem, coincidentally, relates to that yawn Dr. Lima happened to mention: Shift a smidgen on the table and you can create a blur that may look like a blockage. And since you can't have another CT scan for a year, the only way to find out if it's real is to slide an angiogram catheter inside your body. (See "Looking for Trouble" on page 170 for more on the 64-slice CT scanner.)

For now, Hopkins and other top clinics offer patients the less radioactively intense coronary-calcium scan, a quick cardiac CT scan that can pick up unusual plaque deposits along the arterial walls. The calcium scan doesn't show the soft plaque, only the hard, calcified kind that crusts on top of it, but the hard plaque is usually a good indicator of how narrow the artery has become.

"It's exactly the procedure Bill Clinton should have had," says Dr. Blumenthal. "You look at his risk factors when he left office, and he would have been only in the low-risk group. Yet he had three severely narrowed arteries, and the calcium scan would have shown he was at high risk."

## ESCAPING THE MAZE

You're playing hoops, feeling that good burn as your heart rate goes up... and up... and it keeps on going, pounding faster and faster, until it feels as if it's hammering right through your chest. You feel faint, and if you weren't so dizzy, you'd panic. After a few minutes, it passes, leaving you woozy, frightened, exhausted, and wondering what the hell hit you—and when it will hit again.

It wasn't a heart attack: It was the onset of atrial fibrillation, a common condition that can cause the heart to rocket suddenly from 60 beats a minute to 200. The real danger, however, isn't the manic heartbeat, but the silent wreckage it leaves behind. Because the heart is pumping more blood than

**AVERAGE AGE AT WHICH MEN DIE OF HEART DISEASE: 73**

can clear the pulmonary chamber, the excess stagnates, thickens, and can clot in the arteries and choke them off.

More than 1.3 million American men have a-fib, and although the condition is associated with high blood pressure, it's still not known who's at risk, or why. "I've been seeing it hit young, aggressive males—the intense, Wall Street, go-go types," says Charles Mack, MD, whose New Jersey accent and gym-hardened torso make him seem more like a Teamster than a 40-year-old cardiac surgeon at New York Presbyterian Hospital. "They're big-time wine-and-diners who never had a problem before with working hard and partying harder."

Recently, the groundbreaking Copenhagen City Heart Study found scientific proof of Dr. Mack's firsthand observation, showing a connection between a-fib and heavy drinking. And while a-fib strikes many nondrinkers as well, your risk increases significantly if you drain four or more drinks a day. "It's really torture for a young guy—not only does it put him at a high risk of stroke, but it's a horrible blow to his day-to-day life, not knowing when another attack will lay him out," Dr. Mack says. "And if he goes on blood thinners to lower the risk of stroke, sexual performance can go out the window."

Until now, the most effective remedy for atrial fibrillation was a tricky surgical procedure known as "the Maze." Few cardiac surgeons have even learned the technique, since it requires a complex and extraordinarily exact sequence of scalpel slices across the surface of the heart, creating a cross-hatching that looks like a maze. Because a-fib begins with a spasmodic firing of electrical impulses in the upper chambers of the heart, the scars form a series of buffers that act as a sort of roadblock and basically short out the attack before it begins.

"The Maze is very effective but very invasive," says Dr. Mack. "You have to put the patient on a heart-lung machine, stop the heart, and spend a lot of hours in the OR. It's risky."

But recently, two new procedures have been developed that can cure a-fib with fewer complications. First, at the Texas Heart Institute, they're treating the condition with a lassolike device called Ultra Cinch. "You make a small incision in the chest, slide this in, loop it around the left atrium, and hit the juice," says J. Michael Duncan, MD. Embedded in the lasso are pulsers that crackle out ultrasound waves and scar the critical area, much as the Maze does.

"It takes 10 minutes to make the lesions," says Dr. Duncan, one of the first American surgeons to try the technique. He's finding that about 85 percent of his patients are completely cured, and he's also inspired by recent news from Europe that burning a second quick scar into another part of the heart can boost the success rate to as high as 90 percent.

Meanwhile, Sinan Simsir, MD, a cardiothoracic surgeon at Duke University Medical Center, is perfecting a new microwave technique, called the Mini-Maze. Instead of opening the chest and stopping the heart, surgeons enter through small incisions in the sides of the throat. Then they thread in two tiny videoscopes, which allow them to navigate through the carotid arteries toward the left atrium. Once they reach the key section of the heart, they go ahead and scorch it with microwave energy.

"The mortality risk is lowered, since you're not cracking open the sternum," says Dr. Simsir, adding that the procedure also involves next to no recovery time. "In a little while, you're working out again, and you forget you ever had a-fib."

# LOOKING FOR TROUBLE

From EKG to angiogram, here's how our tools for detecting heart disease have evolved.

**Introduced in 1903: EKG.** Short for electrocardiogram, an EKG uses electrodes to pick up each heartbeat's electrical current and display it in a peak-and-valley pattern. It's used while you're at rest or on a treadmill and is often paired with an echocardiogram.
Doctor says you need this test? Be slightly worried.

**Introduced in 1973: Echocardiogram.** High-frequency sound waves are bounced off the heart to produce a moving image of the organ. This echo effect allows doctors to measure the chamber size, pumping efficiency, muscle thickness, and valve operation. Individual arteries and any plaque buildup inside are undetectable.
Doctor says you need this test? Be slightly worried.

**Introduced in 1985: Blood work.** After a close read of the red stuff, doctors can gauge a person's risk of developing heart disease. Levels of two artery cloggers (LDL cholesterol and triglycerides) and one cleaner (HDL cholesterol) are measured.
Does your doctor say you need this test? Don't worry.

**Introduced in 1992: Angiogram.** By feeding radioactive dye into the arteries and then snapping x-rays, blockages can be pinpointed without surgery. If

## THE CONTROL KNOBS FOR CHOLESTEROL

No argument, the best formula for keeping your heart healthy is disciplined eating and exercise. This includes, among other things, seeing trans fats as coronary kryptonite, thinking of saturated fat as only a little less lethal, and breaking a serious sweat several days a week. Oh, yes, and making friends with fiber.

But what if these approaches aren't enough to counter a family history of heart disease, as in the case of 33-year-old Cardinals pitcher Darryl Kile? Is there any surefire way to prevent plaque from clogging your arteries and to blast away what's already accumulated?

If you'd asked 2 years ago, the answer would have been no. But the Cleveland Clinic has tested three new treatments that could "stop heart disease in its tracks," as Dr. Nissen puts it. One, called Reversal, uses high doses of atorvastatin to severely reduce the liver's ability to produce harmful LDL cholesterol.

preliminary blood- and stress-test results are worrisome, doctors will often prescribe an angiogram.
Does your doctor say you need this test? Be very worried.

**Introduced in 1994: Intravascular ultrasound.** This test is similar to the ultrasound used to peek inside a mother's womb, except this procedure reveals the presence of gestating plaque. Doctors snake a catheter tipped with a miniature sound probe into the heart and grab ultrasound images of the artery walls.
Does your doctor say you need this test? Be slightly worried.

**Introduced in 2002: Nuclear exercise stress test.** The name sounds like a reactor meltdown drill, but it's just an EKG, injected radioactive dye, and special cameras that combine to assess heart function at rest and under stress. It allows doctors to spot potential blockages and get a general idea of their locations without surgery.
Doctor says you need this test? Be very worried.

**Introduced in 2004: 64-slice CT:** Only an autopsy is more revealing. After an injection of iodine dye, you slide into a huge, doughnut-shaped device that snaps 64 individual x-rays of your heart in midbeat. These images are then layered together to create a 3-D image that highlights bloodflow and any plaque buildup along arterial walls.
Does your doctor say you need this test? Be very worried.

"The results were striking," says Dr. Nissen, who headed the Reversal trial. "We saw a complete halting of coronary-heart-disease progression in patients who took the high statin doses and continued progression in patients who didn't."

The second therapy is even more exciting: ETC-216, a synthetic form of HDL, was shown in a small study to reduce fatty deposits in the arteries in just 5 weeks. "It was amazing," Dr. Nissen says. "It was the first time anyone showed that therapy could reverse the disease."

Some background: The two kinds of cholesterol in the body—HDL and LDL—are locked in a constant tug-of-war. HDL removes cholesterol from the arteries and flushes it into the liver, but LDL acts in reverse: It's discharged from the liver and into the arteries, where it deposits fatty streaks that can turn into plaque.

ETC-216 is based on apolipoprotein A-I Milano, a unique protein mutation found in only 40 people in the world, the residents of a tiny village in Italy, who have a low incidence of heart disease despite their indulgence in unfiltered cigarettes and fatty foods. When it was discovered that the mutant protein worked by supercharging the villagers' HDL output, researchers came up with the idea of developing a synthetic version. That was 4 years ago.

Clinical trials started in November 2006, and "I've got people calling me all the time asking for it, but there's still a ways to go before it's in your medicine chest," says Dr. Nissen.

But as powerful as ETC-216 is projected to be, it may be overshadowed by an even more effective HDL booster: torcetrapib.

"It literally has cost a billion dollars," says Dr. Nissen. "It's cost more than any other drug to develop. But if the trials pan out, it changes everything."

As Dr. Nissen explains it, torcetrapib has the potential to supercharge the circulatory system to a degree that can't be matched by even the most extensive lifestyle overhaul. "I strongly support responsible lifestyle choices, but there's only so much you can do," he says. "If you combined everything—exercising, losing weight, limiting saturated fats, quitting smoking—altogether, most people would raise their HDL by maybe 5 to 10 percent. Torcetrapib can increase it by 50 to 60 percent!" Just how close is this antidote for atherosclerosis? Pfizer may submit it for FDA approval as early as this year.

## MIRACLE-GRO FOR YOUR HEART

There was no drug in the world that could have helped 70-year-old Nelson Aguia of Brazil. He was in end-stage heart failure, with a coronary muscle so weak it could barely move any blood at all. His doctors told him it was only a matter of weeks, maybe days, till he'd have his final heart attack. But then his daughter, a pediatrician, heard about a radical new experiment being conducted by doctors at the Texas Heart Institute.

Emerson Perin, MD, PhD, director of new interventional cardiovascular technology at the institute, picks up the story. "Let's say you cut your hand—eventually, it repairs itself, right?" says Dr. Perin. "So why couldn't the heart heal itself? When you have a big old heart attack, heart cells die, and you eventually go into heart failure. What we set out to find was some body mechanism that could reverse the damage."

That mechanism is stem cells, which have the chameleon-like ability to mimic whatever new bodily environment they face. Inject them into your brain and they'll start reproducing as cerebral cells; inject them into your quadriceps and they'll replicate into muscle tissue. But the heart—that was a different ball game. "For whatever reason, the repair mechanism you find everywhere else seemed to be overwhelmed in the heart," Dr. Perin says.

But then researchers tried harvesting stem cells from bone marrow in the hip. That did the trick. "The results were amazing," he says. "We took 21 guys who would have died otherwise without transplants, and now they're doing great." The procedure is astonishingly easy: The doctor simply extracts marrow from the patient's own hip, culls out the stem cells that look most promising, incubates them for 3 hours, and then injects them by catheter into the left ventricle of the heart.

"It's like Miracle-Gro for your heart," Dr. Perin exults. One of the original 21 patients happened to die of an unrelated stroke, which gave Dr. Perin a chance to dissect his heart. What he found was better progress than he'd even dared hope for: "His heart was taking on the characteristics of a young, regenerating heart."

In fall 2005 in Houston, Dr. Perin began his second stem-cell experiment to see whether he can duplicate the results of the first. If it goes well, additional trials will be set up at hospitals around the country; if those succeed, a widely accessible treatment should be available in short order.

"When people talk about defeating heart disease," says Dr. Perin, "this is what they mean."

## GUT CHECK

As I traveled across the country, I was given the Idiot Eye by every cardiologist I met. At some point, each would be explaining a complicated procedure and say, "Let's take you, for example. What are your cholesterol and blood pressure?"

"I don't know."

"When was the last time you had a checkup?"

"Freshman year in college—1981."

# ARE YOU HEADED FOR A CORONARY?

We knew stress could strain our hearts, but not like this: A recent study in the *Lancet* shows that stressors such as depression, anger, and anxiety may contribute to heart attacks as much as smoking, obesity, and cholesterol do. To see if you're marked for an infarction, take this test, created by Sheldon Cohen, PhD, head of Carnegie Mellon's Laboratory for the Study of Stress, Immunity, and Disease.

In the past month, how often have you

...been upset because of something that happened unexpectedly?
  A. Never (0 points)
  B. Almost never (1 point)
  C. Sometimes (2 points)
  D. Fairly often (3 points)
  E. Very often (4 points)

...felt you were unable to control the important things in your life?
  A. Never (0 points)
  B. Almost never (1 point)
  C. Sometimes (2 points)
  D. Fairly often (3 points)
  E. Very often (4 points)

...felt nervous and stressed?
  A. Never (0 points)
  B. Almost never (1 point)
  C. Sometimes (2 points)
  D. Fairly often (3 points)
  E. Very often (4 points)

...felt confident in your ability to handle your personal problems?
  A. Never (4 points)
  B. Almost never (3 points)
  C. Sometimes (2 points)
  D. Fairly often (1 point)
  E. Very often (0 points)

...felt that things were going your way?
  A. Never (4 points)
  B. Almost never (3 points)
  C. Sometimes (2 points)

They'd then arch one astounded eye, beaming the unstated but unmistakable question "What kind of idiot are you?" Frankly, it didn't seem all that dumb to me. I run marathons, I hand-saw and split cords of firewood, and my belt has eased out only 2 inches in 2 decades. So why should I worry until I really have something to worry about?

   D. Fairly often (1 point)
   E. Very often (0 points)
...found that you couldn't cope with all the things you had to do?
   A. Never (0 points)
   B. Almost never (1 point)
   C. Sometimes (2 points)
   D. Fairly often (3 points)
   E. Very often (4 points)
...been able to control your irritation with situations in your life?
   A. Never (4 points)
   B. Almost never (3 points)
   C. Sometimes (2 points)
   D. Fairly often (1 point)
   E. Very often (0 points)
...felt that you were on top of things?
   A. Never (4 points)
   B. Almost never (3 points)
   C. Sometimes (2 points)
   D. Fairly often (1 point)
   E. Very often (0 points)
...been angered by things that were outside of your control?
   A. Never (0 points)
   B. Almost never (1 point)
   C. Sometimes (2 points)
   D. Fairly often (3 points)
   E. Very often (4 points)
...felt that difficulties were piling up so high you couldn't overcome them?
   A. Never (0 points)
   B. Almost never (1 point)
   C. Sometimes (2 points)
   D. Fairly often (3 points)
   E. Very often (4 points)

**Scoring:** If you top 12 points, focus on calming down by breathing and talking out your feelings and undergo screening for depression. And work out for 30 minutes a day, 3 days a week; this much sweat can slash depressive symptoms in half.

**PERCENT REDUCTION IN YOUR RISK OF CORONARY DISEASE IF YOU EAT FIVE 4-OUNCE SERVINGS OF FISH PER WEEK VERSUS JUST ONE: 153**

"That's what Chic thought," responded Dr. Blumenthal of Johns Hopkins, "before he died." Henry Ciccarone was a brutally tough player in a brutally tough sport—lacrosse—and even after becoming coach of the Johns Hopkins team, he stayed in peak shape by working out regularly. His parents were healthy into their seventies, which is why Chic was so shocked when he suffered his first heart attack at age 48. After his recovery, he devoted himself as furiously to beating the ailment as he did to beating rival teams, but it was too late—within 20 years, he was dead.

I learn about Chic when I finally show up at Hopkins for my own cardiac screening. They give me the works: First, I stretch out on the table for 10 seconds under the coronary-calcium CT scan to see if I have any hard plaque building up in my arteries.

Then it's up to the exercise lab to find out whether I'm really in the shape I think I am. Exercise physiologist Diana Kuykendall, MS, shaves my wrist and ankle for an electrode body-fat test, which is more exact than using calipers. Then she takes the razor to my chest so she can stick on 10 electrodes for a max-$VO_2$ test, considered to be the best test of overall fitness, since it measures how well your body processes oxygen. She puts a breathing tube in my mouth, clamps my nose shut with a clip, and has me run on a treadmill. The speed and incline gradually increase, until I'm dying for air and have to hop off.

At Texas Heart I get an even more detailed workup. They test my blood for C-reactive protein—a marker of arterial inflammation—triglycerides, LDL and HDL cholesterol, total cholesterol, and fasting glucose. They give me a cup for a protein-in-urine test, pass an ultrasound wand over my carotid artery for signs of plaque buildup, compare my wrist pulse with my ankle pulse, and check my blood pressure.

While waiting for my results, I get a chill of foreboding from William Kraus, MD, an exercise specialist at Duke. "People are deteriorating at a rate that surprises us," he says. "We look at people who should be in the prime of life, and we find deterioration in every parameter: glucose, cholesterol, body size. The national average weight gain is supposedly 1 pound a year, but we're observing 4 pounds a year."

When I get home a week later, all the results are ready. They hit me like a fist in the face. I'd walked into those clinics feeling fit and trim; and now, suddenly, I feel fat and sick. My blood work and blood pressure from Texas check out great, but, according to Johns Hopkins, I have 20 extra pounds of dangerous fat and a low aerobic threshold.

I call Dr. Blumenthal, who explains that the reason the fat doesn't show around my waist is because it's visceral fat, which wedges itself between the organs; but the electrode test caught it. Visceral fat is like a fuel depot for cholesterol, feeding into the liver and spewing back out as artery-choking LDL. "It's the fat you don't see that kills you," he warns.

Even though I've been running and working out, it seems I've gradually let the intensity slide too far into the comfort zone. I never do speedwork anymore, and, come to think of it, it's been 4 years since my last marathon. Just because I look the same on the outside, I've deluded myself into thinking nothing has changed on the inside—where, invisibly, I've actually been subtly deteriorating.

My test results and Chic's story jolt me enough that I buy my first heart-rate monitor and bathroom scale. Instead of just an easygoing sweat, I'm going to make sure my workouts are cranked up into the fat-burning zone. But even though Dr. Blumenthal is glad to hear it, he's not convinced, explaining that the relapse rate after patients receive a health shock is pretty miserable. Dr. Topol has the same gripe: "Once the scare passes, men go back to thinking it will never happen to them."

So for now, I have a reprieve. I noticed my downward slide before it caught up with me. But the real test is still pending: It will be a few years—and a few more mornings in the doctor's office—before I'll know if I've truly taken what I've learned to heart.

# The Search for a Killer

A series of mysterious strokes killed my father. And my grandmother. And two of her brothers. Am I next?

**by William G. Phillips**

There is something oddly comforting about reading my father's autopsy report. Maybe it's the good news: "The skin is normal. The esophagus is without lesions. The stomach is unremarkable. The small intestines contain mostly undigested food particles." Even quitting smoking 17 years before had paid dividends: "There's only mild emphysema."

Or perhaps it's the good that came out of it: "The patient had most organs donated, including kidneys, heart valves, liver, eyes, parts of spleen and lymphatic tissue, bladder, prostate, and most of pancreas."

My father's death, we know from the Center for Organ Recovery, ultimately improved the lives of a half dozen men and women in the Northeast.

Or maybe, probably, it's that it brings me back to the exact moment in time when everything changed. His life, suspended instantly. Mine, altered forever. Yet I feel a sense of potential. Of what might have been had he been holding the railing, as Mom instructed twice. Of how things might have gone differently had we understood what was happening inside his brain that day, or even over the previous 5 years. Or, frankly, if anyone in the family had bothered to wonder what killed his aunt and two uncles, brought his grandmother to stare-into-space dementia, and put his own mother in a nursing home 6 years before, where she lay that fateful day unable to speak or move.

> "The patient lies in bed clutching his abdomen, calling out, 'Help me. Help me.'"—From a memo written by a nurse after visiting my great-uncle George at home in September 1984. He lived like this until he died in January 1991.

I pore through the document over and over, 59 years of humanity summed up and single-spaced on a wholly insufficient five pages, and feel like I'm getting closer. To him. To it—the mystery of what killed him. Because the clinical explanation—"massive intracerebral hemorrhage"—doesn't begin to tell the story. It just deepens a mystery that's three generations old and counting.

My dad fell, backward, down eight stairs. He hit his head on a slate landing. Hard. This opened as many as three dozen bleeding wounds in his brain: hemorrhagic strokes. But it's not that simple. Can't be. Was there a tie-in to those excruciating back pains he'd been having for 3 decades? What about the fact that his right leg would just collapse sometimes? He'd be standing in the middle of the yard and just fall. Was the ministroke he'd had 2 years before a contributing factor? And could it be a coincidence that his uncle George, a decade before him, suffered a parallel set of symptoms and an even more tragic death?

And then, what about this note, buried in my dad's autopsy's addendum: "Findings are consistent with, but by themselves not diagnostic of, CADA-SIL."

What the hell is CADASIL?

Chances are, you know someone who's had a stroke. As diseases go, it's the third-leading killer of men in the United States, behind heart disease and cancer. This year, 700,000 Americans will have one, and a fourth of those will die. Another third will be permanently disabled. And don't think it can't happen to you: One in 12 victims is under age 50, and almost one-third succumb before their work lives are finished.

There are two types. Ischemic strokes, which are caused by a blocked blood vessel, make up around 80 percent of all strokes. Hemorrhagic strokes make up the other 20 percent; they occur when a vessel tears and blood leaks into the brain. My dad's ministroke—diagnosed in March 1997, at age 57, 2 years before his fall—was ischemic. He went to his doctor complaining of lack of balance and of weakness on his right side. An MRI scan revealed a "small infarct" —the stroke—in his left cerebellum, the part of the brain responsible for coordination. But in his medical records, the doctor also noted "moderate lacunar infarcts"—that's doc-speak for a series of so-called silent strokes.

"Most people think of a stroke as a catastrophic event," says David Liebeskind, MD, assistant professor of neurology at the UCLA Stroke Center, the country's foremost stroke treatment and research facility, "but more than 11 million people will suffer a silent stroke this year." That's roughly one in every 25 Americans, mostly men. "A single silent stroke may not cause any symptoms," adds Dr. Liebeskind, "but over time, silent strokes chip away at your ability to function."

It happens when a tiny clot—maybe a piece of plaque that breaks away from a vessel in your arm or leg—meanders to the brain and plugs up a capillary, preventing oxygen-rich blood from reaching the tissue on the other side. Almost instantly, a dime-size part of your brain dies. You, however, feel fine. You don't even know it happened, so you don't change your lifestyle to reduce your risk of another. A couple of years later, it happens again. Then again a few years after that. Soon you can't spin a basketball on your fingertip any-more. Maybe you become frustrated because you keep forgetting the punch line to a joke you've been telling for years. Your balance isn't what it used to be, either, and you can't always find the right word. Suddenly, you're 65 and your grandkids think you're losing your marbles. You actually have been for years, one by one.

"It's called vascular dementia," says Dr. Liebeskind. "It's the second most common cause of dementia, behind Alzheimer's disease. You don't know it's happening until you're older. But if you pulled a hundred 40-year-olds off the street and did MRI scans of their brains, you'd see that a large number have already had a silent stroke."

Maybe that explains why my dad almost drove us off Mount Washington once. It was in 1995, 2 years before he suffered his ministroke. We were above the tree line, heading down; he was driving, I was in the front passenger seat and a vanful of family rode in the back. I noticed that he couldn't keep the vehicle in his lane. Twice, the front wheel edged off the rocky pavement to within feet of the cliff beside me.

"You okay, Dad?" I remember asking.

"Fine," he snapped back. Then, after a pause: "Sure is windy, isn't it?"

It was, and that was that. But my concern crystallized on the 360-mile trip back to New York. I felt like I was riding with someone who'd had one too many. I filed it under "Dad's getting older." I certainly didn't think he might have suffered some sort of stroke. Had he suffered multiple silent strokes before the trip? Doctors can't say; it's impossible to date previous strokes that precisely. But now that I know the signs, I have no doubt.

At the time of his MRI scan, the ministroke diagnosis was actually the good news; it was small and contained, and Dad was already regaining some of the lost function. But his doctor also noticed that the deep center portions of my father's brain showed up as a bright white on the scan. He hadn't seen anything like this before, at least not in a man so young.

These odd images were coming from the tissue—called white matter—that protects nerve fibers. Even more disturbing, large chunks of it were missing. This is not unheard of—white

"I plan to review the records from his family members with strokes, and when testing becomes available for CADASIL, this might be worthwhile."—From the University of Pittsburgh doctor's notes, April 1997. Genetic testing for CADASIL became available in 2000, a year after my father's death.

matter starts developing when you're an infant and slowly begins to disappear in old age. But my dad wasn't old.

Confounded, the doctor referred my father to a neurologist at the University of Pittsburgh Medical Center. Two weeks later, my parents made the 80-mile journey.

My mother drove.

"We should scan your brain."

That was my doctor talking to me 2 months after my father passed away.

"But . . . why?"

"We'll get a baseline," he said. "Then, when you're older, we'll be able to notice any changes in your brain."

"But my father's death was an accident."

"You should have it done," he insisted. "If not right now, then sometime soon."

So I found a new doctor.

I was 29 when my father died. It was the best time of my life, I thought, what with my cool New York apartment, great New York job, and hip New York girlfriend who was taking time off so she could plan our wedding. Sure, my father's death halted my stride a bit, made me think about mortality. But not my own. Despite all the evidence that my dad's fall was caused by something more insidious than a simple loss of balance, for years I referred to his death as a "tragic accident."

Fact is, I probably should have seen it coming the day before the fall.

On October 23, 1999, my fiancée's parents flew in from Milwaukee to meet my family for the first time. They landed at LaGuardia, and we drove them to my sister's place outside of Philly. The women congregated in the kitchen, discussing the rehearsal dinner and the receiving line and ways to turn the hall completely periwinkle. The men hunkered down in the family room, watching the Penn State football team heroically come back and defeat Purdue, 31–25.

We talked fishing, too. Nothing odd here. It was Dad's passion since he'd retired 6 years before. Of course, I use the word *passion* in a relative sense; fishing was one of just two ways my dad passed the time in retirement. The other: sitting in front of the TV, most of the time (thankfully) with it on.

Looking back, this appalls me. My dad once told me, after visiting his own aging father, "If you ever find me sitting in front of the TV day after day like that, promise you'll just shoot me." But it was easy to forgive in my father. Before retiring at age 52, he had spent 17 years, 14 hours a day, 7 days a week, running a small general store in a wilting Pennsylvania town, turning it into a hugely profitable operation. The man deserved a break. He got it with a TV remote, or a rod and reel, in his hand.

He told his fish story that day, and we indulged him.

"So I pulled it in," he said with jerky rod-and-reel hand motions, "and it was another of those damn...ah...those..." He excused himself, went into the kitchen, and quietly asked my mom for the name of the fish he always caught. He nodded and headed back to the family room, but stopped halfway, turned around, and went to Mom a second time. "It's called a crappy," she told him again.

That evening, we all went into town to watch my nephew ride with his Boy Scout troop in a Halloween parade. We parked a few blocks from the parade route. As we walked toward it, my dad was limping, grimacing. During the parade, he leaned against a telephone pole 10 feet behind us. He never saw his grandson ride by. He didn't seem to care.

After the parade, we said our good-byes with no idea of just how final they'd be. My parents left my sister's the following afternoon. On the 4-hour trip home—my mom driving, of course—my dad barely said three words. When they reached home, they entered through the basement. My dad grabbed an overnight bag and started upstairs. My mom was right behind him. On the third step, he fell backward. My mom caught him. "Bill, hold on to the railing," she warned. He didn't respond. On the seventh step, he fell back again. Again, my mom caught and scolded him.

He dropped the luggage in the bedroom and went outside for the mail. My mom started unpacking. A few minutes later, she heard a thud. She ran to the steps. Mail was strewn about. My dad was lying on the landing on his back, legs completely straight, toes up, arms at his sides. This is called posturing; it's a sign of a serious brain injury. He was unconscious but breathing. A rivulet of blood trickled out from behind his head. Mom called 911.

An hour later, around 7:00 p.m., back in New York, my phone rang. It was my sister. "Dad's had a serious fall," she began. "They're flying him to a hospital in Pittsburgh."

My fiancée and I packed quickly and headed for the car. I couldn't bring myself to heed my sister's last piece of advice, so I left my black suit hanging in the closet.

On a cool day in May 2005, I trace that route to Pittsburgh once again. My sense of urgency is different but somehow the same. This time, I'm meeting with Clayton Wiley, MD, the pathologist at the University of Pittsburgh

Medical Center who interpreted my father's autopsy. I get the sense he'd prefer not to be having this conversation but that he acutely understands a son has a right to know.

"Are you squeamish?" he asks me.

"No, not really."

He reaches for his flat-panel computer screen and swings it my way, then double-clicks. A handful of images pop up, each showing a glob of pink tissue and coagulated blood. It looks like nothing in particular—a used placenta, maybe, or a GI's abdomen after a grenade attack—but I know what's coming.

"It's been 2 years and 7 months since George has been in bed. He cannot move any of his body. He has no voice. But he loves to be touched and talked to, even though he can't respond. This gives me hope."—From a letter written by my great-aunt Alice in March 1987

"This is your father's brain."

He pauses to allow it to register, then proceeds: "As you can see, much of the brain tissue has been destroyed. These hemorrhages are not something a person could recover from. The blood clot in the center of the brain alone is 5 inches in diameter.

"Notice how soft the brain tissue is," Dr. Wiley continues. "It's softer than Jell-O. It can't keep its shape. That's an indication that the tissue lacks normal proteins. That it's dead." Of course it is. It's sitting on a table. But I understand his point, that my father was brain-dead long before we pulled him off life support a day and a half after his fall.

Dr. Wiley clicks open another file. "This is a microscopic image of one of the blood vessels in your dad's brain." If not for the purple tinge—dye makes it easier to pick up abnormalities—you could mistake it for a satellite photo of a hurricane. The "eye," just a few microns in diameter, is the blood-vessel cavity. The wall around it is made up of dozens of swirls, as if the vessel were being tied up by kite string. The wall is roughly the same thickness as the hole where the blood is supposed to flow.

"We looked at these vessels because we wanted to see if there was anything in the brain that could explain the severe hemorrhages," says Dr. Wiley. "Blood-vessel walls should be thin. These are extremely thick. And when they're thick, they start to constrict and harden. They'll break like eggshells. This is what happens with hypertension. The vessels are pulsed by high blood pressure, and they thicken to accommodate the increased pressure. That's how high blood pressure causes strokes.

"But your father didn't have high blood pressure, or any of the major risk factors, so something else caused the thickening."

"Something like CADASIL?" I ask.

Dr. Wiley pauses again. "After he died, we did genetic testing for CADA-SIL," he says. "The results were negative. But the tests are only 70 percent sensitive, and we're discovering new variants all the time. I'd strongly suspect CADASIL. Maybe even a variant that hasn't been seen before."

CADASIL is a disease first discovered in a French family in the 1950s. It stands for cerebral autosomal dominant arteriopathy with subcortical infarcts and leukoencephalopathy. In the mid-'90s—around the time of my father's ministroke, in fact—it was linked to mutations in a gene called Notch 3, which lives on chromosome 19. Though the mechanism is unclear, the bad gene causes granules of protein to be deposited in the walls around the brain's blood vessels (and, to a lesser extent, throughout the body). This thickening constricts the vessels and makes them brittle, leading to migraines, mood changes, depression, strokes, and, eventually, Alzheimer's-like dementia.

CADASIL is still considered rare—it's only been diagnosed in about 500 families worldwide—but since the first genetic test became available in 2000, it's been showing up in every corner of the world. "In the end," says Brad Worrall, MD, MSc, assistant professor of neurology at the University of Virginia who's been studying the link between heredity and strokes for 10 years, "it'll probably turn out to be the most common genetic cause of strokes."

The disease tends to appear in middle age: On average, the first symptoms materialize around the age of 45, with the slow mental decline beginning shortly afterward. Most CADASIL patients don't live to 70, though life expectancy varies widely. Even in the same family, says Dr. Worrall, it kills some members in their twenties and others in their nineties.

Dr. Wiley explains that because CADASIL is a so-called autosomal dominant disorder, only one parent needs to have the bad gene for it to be passed on to his or her children. "That means," he explains calmly, "if your father had CADASIL, you have a 50 percent chance of having it, too."

Dr. Wiley senses my discomfort. "But remember, what's true in 2005 may not be true in 2010," he says. "New therapies will come out. If I were you, I'd get a baseline brain scan done. With CADASIL, very specific white-matter patterns show up in MRIs decades before symptoms start, so you'll know right away if you're at risk. And even if it is CADASIL, there may be things you can do to prevent or delay it."

It's the same argument my ex-doctor had made 6 years before, but—

maybe because I'm older, wiser—this time it clicks. I e-mail Dr. Liebeskind for a second opinion. He writes back: "The UCLA Stroke Center is a world-leading institution in brain imaging. I can arrange for an MRI tailored to stroke and cerebrovascular disorders, if you wish."

I book a flight to Los Angeles.

You actually don't have a stroke. You develop one. Meaning: For each minute that passes, a tiny bit more brain tissue dies. This slow progression continues until all the downstream tissue starves to death or the blockage is cleared.

The tissue doesn't die immediately because every major artery in the brain has a few smaller backups, vessels that pick up the slack when another becomes clogged. They're called collateral vessels, and they're the focus of Dr. Liebeskind's research.

The problem with collaterals, says Dr. Liebeskind, is that they're local roads. When a major interstate in the brain becomes blocked, the blood has to turn around, find the appropriate alternative pathway, then take the scenic route to the target destination: brain tissue that's starved for nourishment. This circuitous route, however, largely strips the blood of its oxygen. Even so, the barely oxygenated blood can keep tissue functioning for a few hours; hence, the oft-repeated 3-hour window for reaching a hospital. (Capillaries don't have an effective collateral network, which is why silent strokes kill brain tissue almost instantly.)

Dr. Liebeskind's goal is to find ways to put more oxygen into the bloodstream, then divert more blood into collateral vessels. At Massachusetts General Hospital, doctors have been experimenting with giving supplemental oxygen to stroke victims. "It's quite promising," says Dr. Liebeskind, "but not the complete answer. The route matters, too." So he—along with some of the world's top stroke researchers— is working on therapies that could someday improve an at-risk patient's collateral flow: drugs to make existing vessels larger, for example, or surgery to add new vessels to the brain.

"We've already made huge strides in the past few years," he says. "We're able to bring people back from the brink of death. A person can't speak or walk.

> "His body was donated to Wright State University here in Dayton, and I hope they can learn something about the condition that both Bill and George suffered from."— From a letter written by my great-aunt Mable 2 weeks after the death of her husband, Bill (my dad's other uncle), in April 1995

We go in, open the vessel, and within seconds they can speak and walk again."

The first major advance, a clot-busting drug called tissue plasminogen activator (tPA), was cleared by the FDA in 1996. It's effective at dissolving most clots, but it also has a tendency to cause bleeding in the brain. For that reason, it remains controversial, though a 2004 study found that ischemic-stroke patients who received tPA were twice as likely to recover fully. Still, the 3-hour window is the stumbling block. "Patients are going to the hospital too late," says Dr. Liebeskind, "so only 2 or 3 percent of stroke victims receive tPA."

In 2005, another weapon was added to the neurologist's arsenal when the FDA approved the Merci device, a wire corkscrew developed at UCLA that can be snaked into the brain to remove a clot. There's a lot of excitement around Merci, says Dr. Liebeskind, because it's been approved for use up to 6 hours after the onset of stroke symptoms. "Even in patients where it may have been too late in the past, reopening vessels can improve their long-term outcomes."

Neither of these treatments, however, could have helped my father. "With small-vessel disease, like what your dad had, the only treatment is prevention," says Dr. Liebeskind. "Most strokes, around 60 percent of them, are brought on by high blood pressure, diabetes, high cholesterol, or obesity. The key is controlling your risk factors."

And if you have no risk factors? Like my father, like me? "That's where the other 40 percent come in," Dr. Liebeskind says. "You have to look at genetic factors, which may alter arterial walls or affect the tendency of your blood to clot. We're slowly starting to understand the role of genetics. And once we identify the stroke-causing genes, we can develop specific treatments.

"Decades ago," he continues, "no one thought there was anything you could do about stroke. Today, we're on the verge of major breakthroughs."

Already, says Dr. Worrall, researchers have identified two types of stroke-causing genes. "Probabilistic" genes may increase your risk of stroke, especially if you're exposed to the wrong environmental factors. "Deterministic" genes, it's believed, always cause the disease, though the age of onset varies greatly. Researchers are focusing on probabilistic genes now, because they're more common and some—in conjunction with the right lifestyle choices— also seem to have the power to protect against the disease they cause.

One such gene has been linked to hardening of the arteries. "Preliminary research suggests that if you carry a mutated version of the gene and eat a diet rich in omega-6 fatty acids, your risk is much higher than the general population's," says Dr. Worrall. "But if you eat a diet rich in omega-3 fatty acids, your risk is lower than that of the general population."

Notch 3, the gene linked to CADASIL, is thought to be deterministic, but it has so many mutations that no one knows for sure. Either way, it won't affect the search for a treatment or cure. "The key with CADASIL is figuring out how the bad gene causes the protein deposits," says Dr. Worrall. "If we can do that, we can figure out how to interrupt the process." Several clinical trials in Europe and one in the United States are testing drugs that may do just that.

This knowledge certainly makes the idea of having a brain scan easier to accept, though Dr. Worrall offers a note of caution: "Because your family history is so striking, it's reasonable for you to want to know what your risks are. But we can't treat CADASIL yet. Do you really want to be tested for an incurable, relentlessly progressive disease you have no symptoms of?

"If the test comes back positive, have you thought about how you'll react?"

My brain scan is tomorrow, and I suspect the images will reveal traces of Dr. Worrall lodged in my gray matter.

I can't get him out of my mind—in particular, one theory of medical diagnosis he mentioned.

He described it like this: "In medicine, we always try to explain a set of symptoms with a single cause. If your dad had come to me, I would have looked at the whole picture: the strokes, the white-matter changes, the leg and back pain—his high arches and clawed toes, too, which can indicate an underlying neurological disorder. Then I'd have tried to put it all together with a single diagnosis."

That's exactly what's been bugging me: Nowhere in the medical literature has CADASIL been linked to leg and back pain, though several other disorders do manifest themselves with all of these symptoms. One is CARASIL (cerebral autosomal recessive arteriopathy with subcortical infarcts and leukoencephalopathy), a recently discovered cousin to CADASIL that's inherited only when both parents possess the defective gene. Another is Mast syndrome, a rare type of hereditary paraplegia that my father's uncle Bill was diagnosed with but never actually tested for.

> "Please, no funeral or viewing or obituary! Thanks to each of my family . . . an adventure I wouldn't have missed for anything. So, no tears. Just know I wish each of you joy."—From a letter written to family by my dad's aunt Olive in 1988, months before her first major stroke and 7 years before she passed away

The more I ponder this, the more it feels like I may not know the enemy yet. Suddenly, I can see why Dr. Worrall told me the results of the MRI could be lose-lose.

"What if they spot something and you assume it's CADASIL," he said, "but you end up doing genetic testing and it's not. It's just . . . something. Where do you go from there?

"And what if they see nothing? You think you're free and clear. Maybe you won't watch your blood pressure as closely, or your cholesterol. You're just setting yourself up for a stroke later on."

"What would you do?" I asked him.

"Find out definitively what happened to your dad first," he said. "You mentioned they saved his brain tissue—you can test it for anything. If a relative develops symptoms, maybe he or she can be tested. Once you know what's in the family, then you can decide whether you want to be tested."

A reasonable approach, surely. But in the end, it's my 2½-year-old daughter, Lindsay, who unwittingly seals the decision. She's napping as I pack for Los Angeles. Before I leave for the airport, I wake her up, tell her that Daddy is going away for a couple of days, and hold her close for a few minutes.

I can't help but wonder: Will she have to make a call someday like my sister did, to tell her sister—who will have been born by the time you read this—that Dad's had a serious fall? Will she herself, like my great-aunt Olive, have to write a good-bye letter to family someday in anticipation of a slow, progressive demise?

She looks up at me as I wipe away a tear. "Daddy, will you play with me when you get back?"

"Of course I will, honey."

At that moment, I decide to cancel the MRI. I don't want to come home a different man, a dying man. I will identify the enemy first. Two days later, I have my father's brain-tissue samples sent to UCLA for testing, and, as I write this, the nation's top stroke researchers are on the case. It may take months. It may take years. I will watch and wait.

And live.

# S C I - G U Y

## Protect Your Prostate

Surveying the lifestyles of 1,456 men, researchers at Fred Hutchinson's Public Health Sciences Division in Seattle found that those who drank four or more glasses of red wine per week had a 50 percent lower incidence of prostate cancer than men who consumed less or no red wine. The benefit maxed out at 8 to 14 glasses per week; those men saw a 60 percent reduction in their risk of getting more-aggressive forms of the cancer. This effect may be due to resveratrol, an antioxidant found in the skins of red grapes, which has been shown to block certain enzymes that promote tumor development.

Another study found that soybean-based foods also appear to help the prostate. An Australian study found that men with high levels of prostate-specific antigen (PSA), a possible sign of prostate cancer, experienced a reduction in PSA after eating bread made with soy grits.

## Trade Turf for Surf

Regularly eating one serving of fish per day can cut your risk of developing colon cancer in half, according to a European study of the eating habits of nearly 500,000 people. Researchers aren't sure yet how fish keeps your colon clear of cancer cells, but they speculate that it's not just a matter of substitution. Red meat raises the risk, says study author Elio Riboli, MD, MPH. In the study, people who ate it daily were 49 percent more likely to develop the cancer. A tuna steak probably won't fool you into thinking you're eating a T-bone, but its meaty texture and red flesh make it a good substitute for beef. Grill it to the desired doneness, just like a steak.

## Put Fido to Work

You've heard the stories about dogs sniffing out cancerous growths on their owners' skin. Now, a new study helps confirm the diagnostic prowess of pooches. When British scientists trained six dogs to sniff out cancerous compounds found in urine samples, the dogs were able to correctly identify cancer-ridden samples 41 percent of the time (compared with the 14 percent rate expected due to chance). The dogs also identified cancer in what doctors thought was a healthy sample. While doctors currently have no plans to replace blood work with bloodhounds, they do hope to use canines to learn more about different cancer compounds.

## Ask for Lipitor

Aspirin isn't the only pill that can help you survive a chest-clutching catastrophe. New research shows that swallowing a statin soon after a heart attack cuts the risk of dying in half. A study of 170,000 patients published in the *American Journal of Cardiology* showed that those treated with a statin in the 24 hours following their infarction were 54 percent less likely to die than those not given the drug. "Statins rapidly increase the release of nitric oxide, which has been shown to decrease the amount of heart-muscle damage," says lead study author Gregg C. Fonarow, MD. If you or someone you know suffers a heart attack, ask the attending doctor for a dose of Lipitor (atorvastatin); it's been shown to offer the best protection against heart attacks.

## Eat More Kiwifruit

Scientists at the University of Oslo recently determined that eating kiwifruit may cut your risk of a heart attack. After analyzing blood samples from 30 people who ate two or three kiwifruits daily for nearly a month, the researchers noticed improvement in two important markers of heart disease: Platelet clumping dropped by 18 percent and blood triglyceride levels fell by 15 percent. Though study author Asim Duttaroy, PhD, is still trying to determine how kiwifruits keep us in circulation, he's sure of their benefits. "They should help prevent and protect against the damaging effects of cardiovascular disease," he says. Blend one into your morning smoothie.

## Check Your Heart Rate

Your exercising heart rate can forecast more than calories burned; it can also predict your risk of an early death. French researchers put 6,000 men through a workout, then tracked their health for 23 years. Men whose heart rates rose the least during exercise—by less than 89 beats per minute (bpm)—were six times more likely to die of a heart attack than men whose heart rates skyrocketed. Men whose heart rates didn't drop by at least 25 bpm within 1 minute after a workout also had greater risk of cardiac death. The culprit? A heart that can't adapt to sudden changes in blood pressure, like those that occur during a heart attack, says lead author Xavier Jouven, MD.

## Live to See Another Day

Common prescription medications can stop your heart cold, according to a recent study published in the *European Heart Journal*. Researchers analyzed 775 deaths caused by irregular heartbeats and determined that 41 percent of the fatal arrhythmias were triggered by medications, including the heartburn drug Propulsid (cisapride) and the antibiotics erythromycin and clarithromycin. All the guilty meds have the ability to disrupt electrical activity in the heart, causing long gaps between beats, says lead author Bruno Stricker, PhD. If you have heart disease or a family history of heart trouble, print out the full list of lethal drugs (at www.menshealth.com/drugdanger) and give it to your doctor so he or she can flag your file.

## Bypass the Coffee Shop

Your morning java jolt really starts the blood pumping, but drinking 3 cups of coffee or more each day could cause heart trouble. University of Athens researchers measured coffee consumption and aortic stiffness in 228 people and found that caffeine junkies displayed twice as many signs of abnormal arterial pressure as their less-caffeinated counterparts. "The exact mechanism is not known, but caffeine may interfere with the metabolism of adenosine, a substance that relaxes arteries," says Charalambos Vlachopoulos, PhD. Limit yourself to 2 cups a day, he says. Better still, fill half your mug with decaf, then top it off with regular.

## Juice Up

Recent South Korean research suggests that drinking grape juice can help lower blood pressure. In the study, men who drank two 8-ounce glasses daily for 8 weeks lowered their systolic pressure by 7 points and diastolic pressure by 6—twice the reduction seen in men who drank no juice. Anthocyanins, which are found in grape skin, help dilate blood vessels. Since purple- and red-skinned grapes have the most anthocyanins, choose a dark grape juice.

# Remember Your Pressure

Hypertension drugs may prevent Alzheimer's disease. In a study of 162 people suffering from both conditions, Japanese researchers found that those given the ACE inhibitors Aceon (perindopril erbumine) or Capoten (captopril) experienced eight times less cognitive decline than those given other meds. Researchers say the drugs affect a system in the brain that is crucial for memory but often less developed in people with high blood pressure. If you or your parents have high blood pressure and a risk of Alzheimer's disease, talk to your doctor about these drugs.

# WHAT'S NEW

## LDL-Lowering Lager

They invented the three-point seatbelt, so it's no surprise that Swedes have developed the first beer that can lower LDL-cholesterol levels. The brewing process uses oats instead of barley, infusing the beer with a type of artery-scouring fiber known as beta glucan. Further tests of the beer's effects are under way.

## Sturdier Pills

Are you gellin'? Sometimes you have to have a shot in the arm, especially when stomach acids would make the pill form of a medication ineffective. But soon there may be a way to dodge painful jabs. Scientists in India have developed a gel coating for pills that withstands stomach acid but not the acid in, say, the colon, where the medication might need to be released. Human studies are next.

## Prostate Protection

Men with prostate cancer may soon have a less-toxic treatment option than chemotherapy. In a phase 3 clinical trial, 127 prostate-cancer patients were given injections of either a vaccine, consisting of immune cells and a key cancer marker, or a placebo substance. Three years later, 34 percent of those who received the vaccine, called Provenge, were still alive, compared with 11 percent of the control group. Provenge has been submitted for FDA approval.

Also, Harvard researchers may have found a new way to screen for prostate cancer. After collecting urine samples from 121 men, they tested for

PERCENTAGE OF MEN WHO DON'T HAVE HEALTH INSURANCE: **18**

thymosin beta-15, a cancer marker. Men with prostate cancer and normal PSAs had higher levels. Researchers are honing the test's accuracy to submit it to the FDA.

## Two Strikes against Cancer

Scientists at Israel's Weizmann Institute have developed a way to arm cancer drugs with allicin, a potent antimicrobial compound found in garlic. In a study on mice, the researchers paired the substance with rituximab, an existing cancer-fighting medication. When the dual-action drug reached cancer cells, it destroyed 95 percent of them. If researchers show that the treatment works in humans, it could hold huge cancer-fighting promise.

## Ticker Test

In a study published in the *New England Journal of Medicine*, researchers measured levels of fats called oxidized phospholipids in the blood of 504 people thought to have heart disease. Those with the highest levels were three times more likely to have blocked arteries than those with the lowest. Doctors may be using the test in 5 years.

## One Shot, One Kill

Until recently, surgery followed by 4 to 6 weeks of radiation therapy has been standard operating procedure for treating testicular cancer. Now, a new chemotherapy drug can beat testicular cancer with just one treatment. In a recent study published in the *Lancet*, doctors removed the diseased testicles of 1,477 men and then gave the men either weeks of radiation or a single dose of the chemotherapy drug carboplatin. Three years later, 95 percent of the men in both groups were cancer-free, with the chemo patients reporting fewer side effects. After 5 years, the men given chemo were 72 percent less likely to develop cancer in their remaining testicle than those who'd undergone radiation. In fact, carboplatin might even replace surgery altogether. "This is the first study that suggests that testicle preservation may be an option," says lead author Timothy Oliver, MD.

# T A K E 5

## Avoid the Grim Reaper

Five ways to break your date with death

You're being stalked.

Not by some obsessive ex, who keys your car one day and sends X-rated e-mails the next. Uh-uh, worse. This creep dresses in long black robes and carries around some kind of sharpened farm implement. Goes by the nickname the Grim One. Says he's dying to meet you. Has you scheduled in his BlackBerry.

We advise blowing him off.

Turns out His Grimness sometimes makes it quite clear when—and where—he prefers to collect his corpses. When we analyzed mortality stats and delved into databases about the various and untimely ways young men die, patterns emerged that tip the Reaper's hand.

No, you can't live forever, but by knowing—and avoiding—some of the deadliest times and places in a man's life, you just might be late for your own funeral. (Unless otherwise indicated, all death totals are for men ages 25 to 44, during the most recent year for which data are available.)

**Monday, 8:30 a.m.**
**Location: Your house**
**Death toll: 3,651 heart-attack victims.** Some men make their Monday-morning commute in an ambulance instead of an Audi. After reviewing the hospital records of nearly 5,600 heart-attack patients, German researchers observed that the risk of a heart attack is 33 percent higher on Monday than on any other day, possibly because of the stress of starting the workweek. And in a separate study published in *Circulation*, the deadliest time slot on Monday was found to be the first 3 hours after waking. Why the arterial mayhem in the a.m.? Richard Stein, MD, a cardiologist at New York City's Beth Israel Medical Center, has a good guess: "There's a clear increase in the stress hormone cortisol in the morning, as well as an increased clotting tendency in the blood."

*Survive it:* If you have any risk factors for heart disease—diabetes, high cholesterol, a family history—try to schedule your workout for the afternoon, not the morning. Eric S. Williams, MD, a cardiologist at the Krannert Institute of Cardiology in Indianapolis, says that strenuous physical activity may amplify the effects of the cortisol spike and increased blood clotting. Next, if you aren't already popping a daily low-dose aspirin—81 milligrams—reconsider: Research shows that this regimen reduces the incidence of a morning heart attack by 59 percent. But skip run-of-the-mill pills and instead pick up a bottle of Bayer Low-Dose Children's Chewable Orange; they'll be easier to chew in the event of an actual attack.

**Monday, 11:00 a.m.**
**Location: Your house**
**Death toll: 9,440 suicides.** "Blue Monday" lives up to its billing. Suicides are 10 percent higher on Monday than the weekly average, says John McIntosh, PhD, professor of psychology at Indiana University at South Bend. Using mortality data from the National Center for Health Statistics, McIntosh plotted daily variations in the number of DIY deaths. His finding: "Saturday is the lowest, possibly because there's a buffer from work and stress, and there's self-medication going on. Come Monday, you've gotten through the weekend thinking you'll be better, but you aren't. You have to start this all over again, and you can't take it."

*Survive it:* Are you depressed, and not just because your team tanked in the Sunday-night game? If the answer's yes and you own a gun, lock it up—then throw away the key; firearms are why men are four times more likely

## YOUR TRUMP CARD
### The single most important medical record in a man's life

The average guy's wallet is bursting with all kinds of cards—credit, debit, business, library—but not the one that could save his life: emergency ID. It's the card that, in the event of an accident, will answer all the medical questions you may not be able to, such as "What's your blood type?" "Are you taking medications?" and "Do you have any drug allergies?" Think of it as an EMT cheat sheet. "I've seen many situations in which emergency identification has saved lives," says Ben Abo, emergency-medical-service specialist at the University of Pittsburgh. "Without it, treatment might be delayed." To create a get-out-of-dying-free card, go to www.menshealth.com/MedCard, fill in the fields, hit "Print," cut along the dotted line, and laminate. Then treat your ID like an AmEx card and never leave home without it.

than women to succeed at suicide. Now, see a psychiatrist about taking a selective serotonin reuptake inhibitor (SSRI). In a new study published in the *Archives of General Psychiatry*, researchers said that while antidepressants called tricyclics were associated with higher suicide rates, SSRIs were linked to an overall drop. Also, make sure your multivitamin contains 400 milligrams of folic acid; UK researchers found that folic acid enhances the depression-fighting effect of SSRIs.

**Wednesday, 6:00 p.m.**
**Location: Happy hour**
**Death toll: 259,494 smokers (all men).** If you thought ditching a cell phone carrier was tough, try quitting nicotine. Each year, 35 million Americans attempt to stop smoking; only 1 million succeed. The reasons to quit are powerfully persuasive—dramatic reductions in risk of stroke, heart disease, and certain cancers register within mere years—but logic is no match for tobacco's seduction. "Relapses are most likely to hit in the late afternoon and evening," says Saul Shiffman, PhD, professor of psychology at the University of Pittsburgh's smoking research group. "The classic situation is where there are other smokers and alcohol."

*Survive it:* Nicotine cravings are short-lived, usually lasting 3 to 4 minutes. If you're at a bar (or a party), get through the moment by chugging a glass of water and striking up a conversation with anyone close by, even a complete stranger. "Cold water kills the urge. Talking distracts and delays, and it encourages deeper breathing, which reduces stress," says Alan Peters, MTTS, lead counselor for QuitNet.com. "Try opening a conversation by saying, 'You know, I quit smoking, and right now I'm thinking of having a cigarette.'" And if the person offers you one? Imagine that you-know-who's skeletal hand is proffering the pack.

**Saturday, 1:30 a.m.**
**Location: Multilane roadway**
**Death toll: 10,397.** When the Grim Reaper places an order, he clearly likes it "to go." Motor-vehicle crashes kill more men between the ages of 25 and 44 than any other accidental cause, continuing a trend that begins when guys get behind the wheel in their teenage years. And where, when, and how you drive can significantly stack the odds against you. "Speeding past a bar late at night on the weekend—not a good idea," says Alan Hoskin, statistician at the National Safety Council. In fact, 1,024 sober men were killed by drunk drivers in 2004.

*Survive it:* Rule of thumb: If you have to ask yourself whether you're too drunk to drive, you probably are. Need evidence of your inebriation? Consider carrying the AlcoScan AL5000 (www.alcometers.com), a portable breath-analysis device tested and approved by the National Highway Transportation and Safety Administration.

Or let's say you're driving sober, but the guy coming the other direction isn't, and he veers into your lane. Now what? "Don't bother flashing your lights or honking. You'll only startle him," says Gordon Booth, chief instructor at DriveTrain, a driver-training company in San Jose, California. "Going into the ditch may be your best option. Hit the brakes hard and look where you want to go. Don't fixate on the other car, or you'll unconsciously steer right into him. Even if you put two wheels off the road, that may be enough to get by."

### Sunday, 1:00 a.m.
### Location: Parking lot behind a bar

**Death toll: 6,055 homicide victims.** Saturday night's the night for killer parties, killer dates, and just plain getting killed. Homicide is the fifth leading cause of death among men ages 25 to 44, with business at the morgue picking up on Saturday nights between 10:00 p.m. and 2:00 a.m. "Alcohol and drugs play major roles in high rates of murder on weekends, with arguments and felonies like robbery as the major circumstances," says Kevin D. Breault, PhD, professor of sociology at Middle Tennessee State University. But even if you make it out of the bar or club unscathed, you still have to survive the trip to your car. "You're most likely to be mugged or shot in a parking lot," says Marc MacYoung, crime-avoidance expert and producer of the video *Safe in the Street.*

*Survive it:* Aside from staying ultra-alert as you approach your car, the best way to avoid peril in the parking lot is also the simplest: Spring for valet parking whenever it's offered. Dodging death is a bit more difficult inside a crowded bar, where it's easy to accidentally bump the wrong guy. Next thing you know, he's in your face, veins bulging and fists clenched. What do you do? "Apologize, and mean it. Don't insult him, don't challenge him, don't try a threat display," says MacYoung. "I'd say 999 guys out of 1,000 will accept an apology." If he's the one guy who won't, then just leave the bar. It's really hard to get shot, robbed, or beaten if you're not there.

# MEN'S HEALTH
# QUIZ

## Will You Have Alzheimer's?

Take this quiz before you forget where you put this book

### 1. What would you likely bring to the park?
A. A guitar
B. A picnic lunch
C. A football

Injuries from contact sports are huge contributors to brain diseases, says Daniel Amen, MD, author of *Preventing Alzheimer's*. Playing an instrument is the best hobby for your brain. "Music forces different parts of the brain to work together. Anything that requires coordination and thinking will have the same effect," Dr. Amen says. Try table tennis or chess.

### 2. How do you treat your back pain?
A. I don't have back pain
B. Tylenol
C. Advil

New research shows that constant back pain shrinks your brain. Loss of gray matter in patients with back pain was equivalent to 10 years of aging. Limit the damage by using ibuprofen to dull the hurt. "Tylenol increases your risk of Alzheimer's by inhibiting your liver from producing antioxidants, while taking ibuprofen [for example, Advil] may lower your risk," Dr. Amen says.

### 3. What's your approach to fitness?
A. I try not to approach it.
B. I stick to cardio and weights at a gym.
C. I play sports—the more, the better.

Exercise is crucial to brain longevity, says Dr. Amen, but taking up different fitness activities helps more. "Cross-training stimulates your brain, instead of using the same pathway over and over again," he says. Keeping your weight down is crucial, too. One study found that midlife weight gain doubles the risk of dementia later in life.

### 4. What excites you most about work?
   A. Clocking out
   B. Finding new solutions to problems
   C. Getting to the top of my field

Sure, solving new problems keeps your brain fit. But a study in *Neurology* shows that men who made career strides in their forties and fifties had less incidence of Alzheimer's than those who stayed in the same position for decades. And competitive men climbing the corporate ladder upped the mental demands of their jobs by 33 percent from their thirties to their fifties.

### 5. Which is your strongest sense?
   A. Sight
   B. Smell
   C. Taste

Research shows that people with a keen sense of smell have an advantage against Alzheimer's. In a separate study, declining visual abilities predicted the disease. If you find any of your senses dulling, start taking a multivitamin. A new study found that taking vitamins C and E together lowers the risk of Alzheimer's more than taking them separately.

### 6. Do you drink wine with dinner?
   A. Not usually.
   B. Yes, I often finish the bottle.
   C. I have one or two glasses a week.

Studies show that one or two drinks a week can help your aging brain. People who drank up to seven drinks a week had 7 percent less of a chemical linked to Alzheimer's risk than people who drank heavily (up to four drinks a day). Abstainers had even higher levels. Dr. Amen warns that too much alcohol is toxic to the brain, so don't overdo it.

## PERCENTAGE OF MEN WHO SAY THEY AREN'T AFRAID TO DIE: 60

## 7. Where's your sheepskin from?
A. High school
B. College
C. Graduate school

Another study in *Neurology* reveals that the higher your level of education, the faster your memory loss related to Alzheimer's. Combat it with curry. Researchers at the American Physiological Society recently found that the curcumin in curry stimulates production of the neuron-protective protein hemeoxygenase-1 in your hippocampus.

## 8. What kind of diet are you on?
A. Carbs call my name.
B. A balance of proteins, carbs, and fat
C. High protein

Have a steak. Your brain uses ketones, a by-product of protein metabolism, to protect neurons from free-radical damage. Eat salmon, too. While a low-fat diet has been shown to stave off Alzheimer's, omega-3 fatty acids (found in fish and flaxseeds) protect the nerve-cell connections in your brain against oxidative damage, preserving memory.

### Scoring

| | A | B | C |
|---|---|---|---|
| 1. | A = 3 | B = 2 | C = 1 |
| 2. | A = 3 | B = 1 | C = 2 |
| 3. | A = 1 | B = 2 | C = 3 |
| 4. | A = 1 | B = 2 | C = 3 |
| 5. | A = 1 | B = 3 | C = 2 |
| 6. | A = 3 | B = 1 | C = 2 |
| 7. | A = 3 | B = 2 | C = 1 |
| 8. | A = 1 | B = 2 | C = 3 |

**18 to 24 points:** You'll be telling your great-grandkids details from this article.
**11 to 17 points:** Hope that only the bad memories will fade.
**10 points or less:** Just forget it.

# BURNING QUESTIONS

## Can my cholesterol ever be too low?

Not likely. Although you want your HDL to be high, the lower your LDL cholesterol and triglycerides, the better, says Paul Thompson, MD, director of preventive cardiology at Hartford Hospital in Connecticut. You need some LDL in order to survive. It helps produce sex hormones and build and repair cells, including brain tissue, while triglycerides transport energy throughout the body. But don't fear: According to Dr. Thompson, the only patients he's seen who had unhealthily low LDL and triglycerides were suffering from fatal conditions like lung cancer. Instead of worrying about plunging into a deadly LDL range, focus on bringing your HDL above 45 and keeping your LDL below 100.

## How can I avoid a false hypertension diagnosis?

Pee. "The urge to pee is a terrible stimulus to blood pressure," says Raymond Townsend, MD, a hypertension expert with the University of Pennsylvania Health System. "Holding your bladder stimulates your involuntary nervous system, making you stressed out and thus raising your blood pressure." Most men, thinking they'll have to provide a urine sample at their checkup, arrive for their appointment about to burst. But not you. Call ahead of time to see if a urine sample will be needed; if so, ask to deposit it before you don a BP cuff. Other things to watch for: traffic jams, screaming kids, deadlines, or a cigarette or double shot of espresso in the half hour before your appointment. Even an afternoon workout, if done near enough to the time you're tested, can affect your blood pressure. Try to schedule your test on a low-stress day to avoid scaring up results that will land you on blood-pressure drugs.

## My father recently suffered a stroke. How can I tell if I'm at risk?

Take two tests that gauge the health of your carotid arteries, which supply blood to your brain. The first, a carotid ultrasound test, uses high-frequency sound waves to image these arteries and show plaque buildup. The second, an ankle-brachial index, compares blood pressure in your lower legs with that in your arms to screen for blockages in circulation. (A blockage in one area increases your risk of having one somewhere else.)

"These tests could prevent up to half of all strokes," says William Flinn, MD, vice chair of the American Vascular Association (AVA). If a blockage is found, you can control it with drugs, diet, and exercise. "Unfortunately, we have a reactive health-care system in this country, not a preventative one," says Dr. Flinn.

Neither test is covered as a preventive measure by private insurers or Medicare, but you can get them for free at AVA-approved screening centers. Call 877-282-2010 or visit www.vascularweb.org.

### My father developed degenerative arthritis in his spine as he got older. Is there anything I can do to avoid the same fate?

There's one surefire method: Bend at your knees, not at your waist, when you lift heavy objects. "Most people bend at the waist, which places undue stress on the lower vertebrae and disks," says Ellis Friedman, MD, author of *Outwitting Back Pain*. "Over time, the edges of the vertebrae grow larger to spread that stress across a greater surface area." The result is degenerative arthritis.

Proper technique also entails keeping your body straight and taking a deep breath as you lift. "The deep breath will tighten your stomach muscles and increase the force on your abdominal cavity," says Dr. Friedman. "In effect, you'll be turning your torso into a hydraulic cylinder, which will take some of the weight and pressure off your spine." For added insurance, Dr. Friedman recommends strengthening your abdominal and lower-back muscles.

### The latest news reports about vitamin E have me scared. I've been popping it since college. Have I been setting myself up for a heart attack?

The jury is out, but it's leaning toward no. The study behind the recent reports comes from Johns Hopkins University, where researchers found a 5 percent increased risk of death among subjects who took more than 400 IU

**PERCENTAGE OF AMERICANS WHO DON'T REALIZE THAT BEING OVERWEIGHT PUTS THEM AT RISK OF DEVELOPING DIABETES: 59**

of vitamin E per day. But for proper perspective, you need to consider who was studied: All of the subjects were older than 47, and the majority of them had preexisting medical conditions, such as heart disease. The USDA recommends a more conservative daily allowance of vitamin E: 22.5 IU, or 15 milligrams. The average adult male gets half of that from dietary sources such as nuts and green leafy vegetables. You can also hit the recommended mark with a multivitamin; most contain about 30 IU of E.

### I quit smoking, but now I'm addicted to nicotine gum. Am I just as bad off as I was before?

No. Cigarette smoke contains more than 60 carcinogens and 4,000 chemicals, including arsenic. The gum contains only nicotine. While studies have linked this chemical to increases in both heart rate and blood pressure, the quantity you get from chewing the gum is very small (about a third of what you'd receive from a cigarette), according to Richard Hurt, MD, director of the Mayo Clinic Nicotine Dependence Center in Rochester, Minnesota. "Still," says Dr. Hurt, "there could always be side effects we don't know about yet."

When you're ready to quit, begin with a slow taper. Dr. Hurt recommends chewing one less piece every week. Use the 4-milligram-strength gum if you smoked 25 or more cigarettes a day or the 2-milligram-strength gum if you smoked fewer.

To get the most out of the gum (and cushion the blow of withdrawal), "bite it a few times and park it between your gum and your cheek," says Dr. Hurt, explaining that absorption takes place through the lining of your mouth. For more information, go to www.mayoclinic.org/stopsmoking.

### My prescription has a warning label about grapefruit juice. Why shouldn't I drink it with my meds?

Grapefruit juice affects the action of two key enzymes in the liver that are responsible for metabolizing a wide range of medications. "In the case of VePesid [etoposide, a cancer drug], metabolism is increased, causing it to disappear from the body faster than normal and thus not have the desired effect," says Amy Karch, RN, MS, an expert on drug interactions at the University of Rochester Medical Center in New York. "With Viagra [sildenafil citrate], on the other hand, metabolism is lowered, leading to increased [and potentially toxic] levels of the drug in the body."

Since grapefruit juice doesn't interact directly with the drugs but rather influences a bodily process, its effects can be felt long after you take your last sip. "It can take up to 48 hours to clear the chemicals in the juice from your body," says Karch. Bottom line: If the label warns against grapefruit juice, switch to orange.

## Is constant low blood pressure a bad thing?

You probably have nothing to worry about, says *Men's Health* cardiology advisor P. K. Shah, MD. In general, low blood pressure is a good thing in otherwise healthy people. Well-conditioned athletes often have low readings. But feelings of weakness could be a sign that your blood pressure is too low. If you often feel light-headed when you get dehydrated, you should see your doctor.

## I'm 30. Am I safe from testicular cancer?

Nice try, but you're never off the hook, says *Men's Health* urology advisor Jon Pryor, MD. It's true that it's considered a young man's disease, and it's unlikely after age 35. But you can still get it, even as an old man. Continue monthly self-exams in the shower, when your scrotum is soft and lumps are easier to detect. If you feel anything new, see your primary-care physician or a urologist.

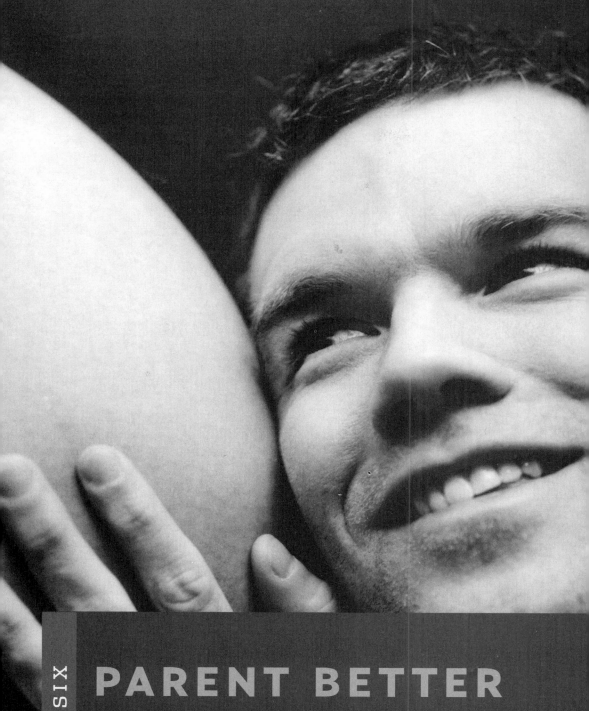

SIX

# PARENT BETTER

# READ UP ON IT

## My Advice: Tim McGraw

"Fatherhood changes you. It's in your whole being, in your soul."

### Interview by Mike Zimmerman

Every man hates his father at some point—usually when Dad is being too much of a dad: the hard-ass, the hard-hearted, the disciplinarian. But the damage runs deeper when Dad isn't being a dad at all. Country-music super-star Tim McGraw, 37, knows that firsthand. When he was a boy, his father, baseball legend Tug McGraw, refused to acknowledge him as his son. (Tug had a brief encounter with Tim's mom back when Tug was in the minors.) Even after Tim and his dad met, in 1979, it took many more years for Tug to warm to the idea of having a son. Eventually, though, the pitcher stepped up to the plate. As adults, both men committed to finding what was worthwhile in their relationship, until Tug's death from brain cancer in January 2004. Now, as Tim raises three children of his own (all girls) and manages a block-buster music career (his album *Live Like You Were Dying* memorializes Tug), he offers some hard-won wisdom on dealing with your father—while trying to become a better one yourself.

**On getting over hard feelings toward your dad.** "I don't think Tug was ever trying to do the wrong thing. As he and I got older, we became closer and closer, but I don't think we ever had a father-son relationship. It was more like uncle-nephew. Unless, some of the time, I was the father and he was the son [laughs]. The main thing I took from all those years is an understanding: Basically, people are trying to do the best they can, no matter what it looks like to everybody else. They're working with what they have, and some people just don't have the tools to do the things that we think they ought to be doing. That was the case with my dad."

**On recognizing your own power.** "All kids expect a lot out of their par-ents, but you have to expect more out of yourself. See, even though Tug didn't acknowledge me growing up and turned his back on me when I first sought him out, I still developed an inner drive and confidence because my father was so successful at what he did. That made me feel like I could be successful at anything I wanted to do, too. But Tug couldn't do it for me. I had to go out and do that myself."

**On becoming a great father when your own father wasn't so great.** "Filling that void I had growing up certainly had something to do with my wanting to be a dad. I always knew I wanted kids. If I could've gotten away with it, I would've had kids when I was 16. But that's probably why I didn't get married until I was 29. I wanted to raise my kids right. I wanted to be able to take care of them, to be stable, and to just plain be there for them. So in a way, without even knowing it, Tug gave me the tools to be a great dad."

**On why every man needs to become a father.** "People can tell you that fatherhood changes you, but you just don't have any idea. It's a change in your whole being, in your soul. It changes your capacity to love, even the way you love everything else—your country, your world, your god, your wife, your friends. Realistically, it's not that far from being saved, because in a lot of ways that child is your eternal life."

**On the temptation to be superdad.** "There's going to be a broad gap between your ideal of yourself as "the father" and the real, flawed human being that you actually are. And the person who has to know this best is you, the dad. I constantly battle myself: Am I doing the right thing? Should I do this? Should I not do this? It's a daily perplexity. It's always there. So you have to look in the mirror and not beat yourself up about the decisions you make. You can't be a perfect parent. You just can't [smiles]. Doesn't mean you can't try, though."

**On the one area, above all, where a father cannot fail.** "Not being there is the biggest mistake a father can make. And I don't just mean physically. I mean not being there. Not being present. Do this right and you can be gone for a week and your kids will still know that you're there. You can be divorced and your kids will still know that you're there. You'd like to think that your kids can feel you hugging them their whole life, no matter where they are. You fear for them, especially with girls. But maybe if you can give them that presence, that feeling that you're with them all the way through, then if something bad ever does happen to them, at least they knew that you were there. [pause] Man, I hate even talking about that."

# McGRAW'S MANDATES

**1.** Forgive your old man. He did the best he could.
**2.** Even your failures can teach your kids a lot.
**3.** Fatherhood transforms a man, so welcome it (when you're ready).
**4.** When you're with your kids, really be there.

# Words of Wisdom

You might not believe it until they've grown up, but your kids really are
paying attention

**by Roxanne Patel**

Harry Truman's daughter, Margaret, once said about a woman's relationship
with her father: "It's only when you grow up, and step back from him, or leave
him for your own career and your own home—it's only then that you can
measure his greatness and fully appreciate it." Maybe your dad never rose to
that level of "great." Maybe he spent more time fixing the blasted lawn mower
or repacking the family car for that trip to the shore than he did bargaining
with Stalin and Churchill about the fate of the world. Even so, we're betting
the man you call Dad passed along some nuggets of knowledge about the
world that still live on in your heart and mind. Here, from the mouths of
women famous and not so famous, are some fatherly lessons that have survived the test of time—not to mention a few family road trips.

"My dad fathered by leaving us on our own. If I got in trouble, he made
me figure out how to get out of it myself. I was always bitter about that. But
now I realize it's helped me—I'm a survivor because of it."
**Denise, 36, marketing director**

"My dad showed me how to roll pennies. First you stack them in piles of
10. Then you stick the tube on your index finger and put the coins in the
top, 10 at a time, inching your finger down until it's at the bottom of the
tube. That way they don't tip to the side. I'm still convinced it's the only way
to do it."
**Vicki, 34, editor**

"My father was very strong. I don't agree with a lot of the ways he brought
me up. I don't agree with a lot of his values, but he did have a lot of integrity,
and if he told us not to do something, he didn't do it either."
**Madonna, singer/actress**

"My dad taught me the only way to make a vodka tonic—when I was 5:
Fill a tall glass all the way with ice. Pour in a shot of vodka; fill the rest with
tonic. Squeeze a slice of lime and a lemon, then drop them in the glass. And
finally, this is key: Stir with the same knife used to cut the lime and
lemon."
**Sara, 23, editorial assistant**

"I just owe almost everything to my father, and it's passionately interesting for me that the things that I learned in a small town, in a very modest home, are just the things that I believe have won [this] election."
  **Margaret Thatcher, upon being elected UK prime minister**

"My father is an electrical engineer and I was brought up paying a lot of attention to how things work. When the refrigerator door wouldn't close, you didn't just keep shoving and slamming it; you opened it further and examined everything that was in the path of the door, as well as its hinge. It was a real object lesson in gentleness, as well as a very practical way to learn how to get the most use out of your material possessions."
  **Liesel, 34, actress/musician**

"My father tried to teach me how to do a headstand. That resulted in me not being able to walk for a week."
  **Camille, 31, florist**

"My dad told me you can stick with any job for 6 months. If it's not the experience you expected, chalk it up to a lesson learned and move on."
  **Alison, 34, marketing brand manager**

"My father taught me not to be so serious. I went to an all-girls school and had to wear a blue and gray uniform. On St. Patrick's Day in third grade, my dad told me to wear green tights to school. I refused, because it was against the rules. He kept insisting; I kept saying no. Finally, he paid me $20 to wear the tights. All the fourth- and fifth-graders thought I was totally cool for doing my own thing."
  **Ann, 26, entrepreneur**

"My father decided I was ready to start tennis lessons when I had just turned 5. I used his old wooden tennis racket, and every Saturday he threw tennis balls at me for hours, hoping one of my many swings would actually hit the ball. This went on for years, and we moved on to basketball, softball, and volleyball. By the time I was in third grade, I was on every sports team the school had, even beating boys my own age."
  **Natalia, 34, graduate student**

**POSSIBLE PERCENTAGE REDUCTION IN HEALTHY SPERM FROM CARRYING A CELL PHONE IN YOUR PANTS POCKET: 30**

"My dad taught me how to drive in reverse. He made me drive from the beginning of our development, around a big curve, up a hill, into our circular driveway, through two narrow stone walls, down a path, and into my garage space—all backwards. After that, I never once got confused about which direction the ass of my car would go when I turned my steering wheel."
**Carrie, 23, editor**

"I worked hard and made my own way, just as my father had. And just, I'm sure, as he hoped I would. I learned, from observing him, the satisfaction that comes from striving and seeing a dream fulfilled."
**Sigourney Weaver, actress**

"My father forbade food dares at the dinner table. While I always thought it was stupid when I was young—why shouldn't I eat a tater tot dipped in peanut butter if I want to?—I now see the logic behind it all. Food dares lead to bigger dares—drinking dares, drug dares, and worse. Learning to say no when I was little was good practice for when I was older and faced with bigger obstacles."
**Rachel, 23, marketing coordinator**

"My dad told me not to grab a salamander by the tail. He said, 'Go for the head, because if you grab it by the tail, the tail could come off. And the tail, if it falls off, may still wiggle around on the ground.' I always remembered that and managed never to pick up a salamander by the tail."
**Heather, 33, stay-at-home mom**

"It doesn't matter who my father was; it matters who I remember he was."
**Anne Sexton, poet**

"My father told me if you eat all the candy inside the store it's not really stealing."
**Melissa, 28, fashion buyer**

"My dad is famous for saying, 'Why save dessert until the end of the meal?' They're words to live by."
**Becky, 35, publicist**

# Kid Control

10 ways to keep your kids in shape

**by Jamie Bellavance**

It may be tough to tell junior that he's packing on the pounds. Odds are, the child already knows that he or she is overweight, has been ridiculed by peers at school, and needs a parent to step in and take action. We talked to experts about easy solutions parents can use right now to help the husky.

**Work together.** "Tell them you love them the way they are but that you need to be healthy together," says Valerie Mokides, DO, an osteopathic pediatrician in New Hyde Park, New York. Start exercising together, go for walks together, and play a part in his or her after-school activities or sports. "Support what they're doing and cheer them on," she says.

**Be a positive example.** The parent is the child's first teacher. If Daddy works out in the gym, the child will want to look like Daddy. "Parents need to be a role model—keep in shape and eat healthy—because that's where kids learn most of their habits," says John Whyte, MD, vice president for the Discovery Health channel.

**Beware of beverages.** Water and juice should be a child's main beverages. But watch out for some juices that pack more sugar than soft drinks. "The label should say 100 percent natural or 100 percent juice. There is no need for sugar in fruit juice," says Dr. Mokides. Also watch children's soft drink intake, especially while at school.

**Ban bad beverages.** Parents can even request that schools eliminate or cut down on soft drink vending machines present on school grounds. Some schools have adopted antisoda guidelines, so contact your local school board to find out what can be done.

**Everything in moderation.** Be conscious of how many calories your child is eating and balance it with activity. "It's not about denial," says Dr. Whyte. "It's about balance." For every hour spent in front of the TV, do some

**PERCENTAGE OF MEN WHO BELIEVE HAVING KIDS IS VITAL TO "THE GOOD LIFE": 76**

form of activity. During commercial breaks, make a contest out of who can do the most pushups or jumping jacks.

**Keep fruits and veggies in the open.** Fruits and vegetables are the original fast food. Bury the tempting cookie jar and replace it with a bowl of fresh fruit from which children can self-serve. Pack a snack bag for the road to avoid resorting to fast-food restaurants when the kids are hungry. There should be no excuses for using the drive-through for a quick bite to eat when it takes less than 5 minutes to eat a piece of fruit.

**Walk it off.** Meet your child a few bus stops earlier than usual and walk together. Another idea—when you go out with your child, park the car far from the building and walk, then take the stairs instead of the elevator.

**Make a substitution.** Cook your usual meals, but play with the ingredients. Use less butter and oil. Substitute lower-fat ingredients like reduced-fat cheese, low-fat or fat-free milk, and lean meats. No one will notice the change if you gradually use healthier ingredients.

**Practice portion control.** Use smaller plates to serve meals, so portions look larger. Order a medium pizza instead of a large. Everyone still gets the same number of slices, but the slices will be smaller.

**Dine out smart.** If a restaurant fails to offer a healthy option, don't be afraid to ask for a vegetable instead of french fries or pasta. Split an entrée with your child and order a salad on the side. Keep that in mind with dessert, too. It's okay to want a cookie, but if your child's going to have one, make sure he or she shares half with a buddy.

# SCI - GUY

## Butt Out

Smoking has already been linked to impotence, and new research shows that it affects sperm production, too. A study published in the *Journal of Clinical Endocrinology & Metabolism* showed nicotine inhibits the secretion of luteinizing hormone, which stimulates production of testosterone and sperm. The effect disappeared within 1 week of quitting.

## Blame Your Genes

Male fertility problems can be genetic, says *Men's Health* urology advisor Larry Lipshultz, MD. In a screening of men with severe fertility problems, 25 percent showed an abnormality in genetic tests. Most of these men have problems with sperm production. A genetic evaluation would include a close examination of the Y chromosome to look for missing parts.

## Breathe Easier

Smog may affect your swimmers, according to a new report in the journal *Environmental Health Perspectives*. Analysis of more than 5,000 sperm donations over a 2-year period in Los Angeles revealed that when ozone levels increase, sperm concentrations decrease. "If you're trying to get your partner pregnant, don't go outside to do intense physical activity when the temperature and air-pollution levels are high," says Rebecca Sokol, MD, professor at the University of Southern California. The report speculates that ozone causes oxidative stress, which is known to disrupt testicular and sperm function.

**COST OF RAISING A CHILD TO AGE 18:**

**$170,460**

## Time It Right

A new study of 86,436 U.S. births shows that there is a slightly increased likelihood that women who are married or living with a man will have sons. Researchers say it may have to do with the timing of intercourse. Sperm with the manly Y chromosome are more likely to outswim the Xs early in the fertile window—1 to 5 days before ovulation. Cohabitating couples may be having "fruitful intercourse" earlier than those not living together, speculates Karen Norberg, MD, of the National Bureau of Economic Research.

## Save on Braces

An Italian study shows that breastfeeding leads to straighter teeth than bottle-feeding. Nursing encourages proper development of the palate and mouth muscles, which protects against the tooth-moving effects of thumb sucking.

## Blame Mom

If a plate of brussels sprouts triggers your gag reflex, blame your parents. English researchers monitored 40 infants over a period of 2 years and learned that babies who are introduced to a wide range of new foods in the 1st year of life will happily eat them later. By age 2, young 'uns recognize the look and feel of foods that they've eaten before but refuse those that fall into the "unknown" category.

## Ask for the Kids' Menu

Child-size portions keep kids from overeating, according to a new Cornell University study. Kids eat what's in front of them, researchers found; hunger has little effect on calories consumed.

## Play Around

Here's a great twofer: Be a good dad and get a good workout. Playing with your kids can be as beneficial as certain workouts, according to a new study in the *Journal of Sports Medicine and Physical Fitness*. Just 20 minutes of playing soccer and dodgeball raised adults' heartbeats to 88 percent of their maximum and burned 160 calories, researchers found; half an hour burned 240 calories—about the same as a moderate bike ride. The games were more than enough "to produce training effects and benefits from physical activity," says study coauthor Phillip Watts, PhD, of Northern Michigan University.

## Check Up

A study at St. Louis University found that only 53 percent of dads regularly go along on doctor visits. Be one of them and you'll learn about immunizations and allergies—information that could save your child's life in an emergency, says study author Trevena Moore, MD. Plus, a scary doctor's or dentist's office is a chance to talk about fears, making it easier for your child to turn to you in trying times, says Ronald Levant, dean of psychology at Nova Southeastern University.

# WHAT'S NEW

## Preggers Protein

Japanese scientists say they've found the protein in sperm that allows it to fertilize eggs. The discovery could be helpful in birth control and in the treatment of infertility, according to their report in the journal *Nature*. Sperm from mice without the protein could not bind to an egg to fertilize it. The researchers named the protein "izumo," after a Japanese shrine to marriage.

## Super Scrubber

Get your kids to fight over cleaning the bathroom. Buy a Black & Decker S600 ScumBuster cordless scrubber (about $40, www.blackanddecker.com). Your kids will be jockeying for bathroom-cleaning duty for the next 6 months. "Let's face it," says Dan Warlick, a father of two boys in Durham, North Carolina. "Put a motor on something, and guys of all ages will love it."

## A Rose by Any Other Name

Women are increasingly taking their husbands' last names. Only 17 percent of American women keep their surnames after marriage, according to a University of Florida study. Diana Boxer, PhD, linguistics professor and study author, says her study reflects a reversal of the trend of the 1970s through 1990s, though comparable statistics are scarce. The name choice doesn't have to happen before the wedding, she notes. Successful career women may be reluctant to make a change, "so the decision can come when children are born," says Dr. Boxer. Whatever the inclination, she advises that you "discuss it frankly and come to a joint decision."

**PERCENTAGE OF KIDS WHO WISH THEIR FATHERS WOULD SPEND MORE TIME WITH THEM: 40**

# The Ultimate Tree House

Soccer games and sundaes fade like all the other ephemera of childhood. Want to make a lasting impression on your kids? Follow these tips to build them an unforgettable backyard retreat.

1. **Choose your tree.** One-tree roosts require 6-inch or larger trunks; smaller limbs call for grouped stands.
2. **Plan your project.** The tree is your architect: Its vagaries determine your layout. Hone your blueprint using plans you'll find on www.treehouseguide.com.
3. **Build your foundation.** Use Garnier Limbs (www.treehouses.com), not nails—these bolts boost load-bearing capacity to 4,000 pounds.

# T A K E  5

## Decipher Teen-Speak

### Five ways to avoid a communication breakdown

Don't spend your child's adolescence walking on eggshells. Instead, try these five methods to connect with the creature that dwells behind the Jessica Simpson poster–covered door.

**Listen up.** "Whatever!" Door slam. If this combination of dialogue and stage direction plays regularly at your house, you're probably making the common parenting mistake of talking twice as much as you're listening. "Lecturing is the easiest way to get a teen to shut down," says Ken Canfield, PhD, president of the National Center for Fathering.

**Give intimacy to get intimacy.** If asking what's troubling your teen is met with a dismissive "nothing," offer a personal anecdote, but avoid saying "when I was your age." It's the conversational equivalent of elevator music.

## THE TEEN TRANSLATOR

The culture of adolescence has its own language. Here, clinical psychologist Nancy Molitor, PhD, breaks down some common phrases.

| What He Says | What He Means |
|---|---|
| "I'm fine." | "Your question is simplistic and I can't be bothered to answer it." Instead, ask, "Anything bum you out today?" |
| "Not now." | "I want to be in charge, so I'm defining when we'll talk." Find out if your son has time to go out for ice cream. |
| "Whatever." | "I don't know how I feel or what to say—I'm buying time." Or, he finds your question annoying. |
| "I hate you." | "I'm angry." (If he hates you, he won't say.) Ask why he's angry. |
| "You suck." | A more profane version of "I hate you." To keep your son from using coarse language at home, declare the house a no-swear zone—and then abide by your own law. |

Instead say, "I might not understand what it's like to be 15 today, but I do know about loneliness."

**Criticize the behavior, not the child.** Say "I'm angry that you're making bad decisions" instead of "Only losers smoke pot." Your son will understand he has control over his actions, according to Marc A. Zimmerman, PhD, professor of psychology at the University of Michigan.

**Look for teachable moments.** Let an event be the catalyst for a big talk. If your daughter's thumbing through a supermarket tabloid and says, "Lindsay Lohan has so many boyfriends," that's a segue into a discussion about sex. Getting on neutral turf outside the house—where you as parent are in control—also encourages conversation.

**Don't be a ghost.** When a teen tells you "Go away," it means "Leave me alone for now, but check on me." Show your daughter you care from a distance by slipping a note under the door, one that reminds her how much she means to you. "If you back off too much, you're not going to know what is important to her," says Nancy Molitor, PhD, assistant professor of psychiatry and behavioral sciences at Northwestern University Medical School. And when you do finally have a sit-down, let your daughter know she's your number one priority by turning off your cell and PDA.

# MEN'S HEALTH QUIZ

## Are You a Good Dad?

Take this test to find out if you deserve your Father's Day card

**1. How many friends do you have?**
   A. I've got a few, but they're good ones.
   B. Tons—people are always coming by.
   C. Do pets count?

Social dads raise kids with fewer behavioral problems, according to researchers at King's College in London. But only if their circle includes other dads and provides affirmation at important milestones in a child's life, says Jeff Evans, PhD, JD, researcher at the National Institute of Child Health and Human Development.

**2. Have you found religion?**
   A. Never lost it.
   B. Nope, and I'm not looking.
   C. Not really, but I go through the motions.

Religious dads are typically more involved with their children than nonreligious fathers are, according to a study from Pennsylvania State University. Religious or not, follow your own gospel, says Greg Lang, author of *Why a Daughter Needs a Dad*. Kids always see "inconsistencies between how a parent says a child should act and how the parent acts," he says.

**3. You'll be there for them most during . . .**
   A. Infancy
   B. Childhood
   C. Adolescence

It's not enough to provide the blueprint for success, says Dr. Evans. You have to make sure the building goes up right. "A dad's role in his child's transitions is crucial and requires being there beyond the first few years of life," he says.

You can't ask the tough questions until they can talk, says Roland Warren, president of the National Fatherhood Initiative.

**4. Your discipline philosophy is . . .**
A. Let the punishment fit the crime.
B. Let the punishment fit the child.
C. Let them do whatever they want.

Dads tend to be the enforcers. But successful discipline means tailoring the punishment to the child, Warren says. Go with whatever method gets results with each child. Remind your kids soon after meting out punishment why their actions led to it. Then explain that your relationship will never change and that your love for them is unconditional.

**5. What does the playroom look like?**
A. My whole house looks like a playroom.
B. A Toys "R" Us explosion
C. Colorful, neat, and organized

Kids need sane, hazard-free homes (and you deserve a neat refuge), but they also need to indulge their creativity, says Gary Greenberg, author of *Be Prepared: A Practical Handbook for New Dads*. Let them reign over one room. "Lay mats on the floor, put giant reams of paper on the walls, and save cleanup for when every inch is covered," he says.

**6. You and the kids' mom are . . .**
A. Loving and committed
B. Miserable and contentious
C. Friendly but unromantic

Happily married couples tend to make the best parents, but happily divorced parents aren't far behind. Whether you're divorced or not, one of Dad's most important functions is as "a support system to Mom," says Dr. Evans. After a

PERCENTAGE OF DADS WHO GO OUTSIDE
TO PLAY WITH THEIR CHILDREN AT LEAST ONCE
A WEEK: 68

divorce, many kids think their dads become more attentive and involved in their lives, Dr. Evans says.

**7. "Quality time," to you, means . . .**
   A. Reading them two books before bedtime
   B. Soccer at 9, karate at 12, violin till bedtime
   C. Any time is quality time

"Kids work from the perspective of 'This is what's happening now,'" Warren says. "If you don't have quantity time with kids, you can't have quality time." Big questions and problems come up unexpectedly, so be flexible. Resist over-planning, Greenberg says: "Staying home and playing fort is often more fulfilling than a day of scheduled activities."

**8. Your fatherly lesson plan starts with . . .**
   A. Finance 101
   B. Algebra, grammar, and history
   C. Learning to ride a bike and throw a curveball

"What men do best is play with their kids," Dr. Evans says. "You can encourage your children to be daring, reassure them of your presence, and convey a mindset toward life, all through play." Sports will stimulate your children to be more active, to respect rules, and to work with others, which will keep them healthier throughout their lives.

## Scoring

| | | | |
|---|---|---|---|
| 1. | A = 3 | B = 2 | C = 1 |
| 2. | A = 3 | B = 2 | C = 1 |
| 3. | A = 1 | B = 2 | C = 3 |
| 4. | A = 2 | B = 3 | C = 1 |
| 5. | A = 1 | B = 3 | C = 2 |
| 6. | A = 3 | B = 1 | C = 2 |
| 7. | A = 2 | B = 1 | C = 3 |
| 8. | A = 1 | B = 2 | C = 3 |

**18 to 24 points:** Hoist that World's Greatest Dad mug with pride.
**11 to 17 points:** Focus more on your family; they need you.
**10 points or less:** Know your local police? You will soon.

# BURNING QUESTIONS

**If you were to choose just one piece of advice to give fathers, what would it be?**

Become a better husband. It's your most important job. Fatherhood is your second, and it will fall right into place if you have a deep respect for your wife and you display that respect in front of your children. Men can be self-centered. Be aware of the needs of other family members, especially your wife. Work on your coparenting skills. Different perspectives on disciplining kids create most of the major conflict and tension in families. Want to fix that? Have weekly "executive team" meetings with your wife to address time-management, school, and health issues. Also, make time for just the two of you. Kids are guests; you two are forever.

**My wife and I are in our thirties but don't want to have kids yet. How late is too late?**

For a general idea of the absolute latest you can conceive, use this equation developed by Cara Birrittieri, author of *What Every Woman Should Know about Fertility and Her Biological Clock*. Subtract 10 years from the age at which her mother hit menopause. (Have her do the math; there are some things a man just shouldn't ask.) Subtract 2 years if your wife smokes, 6 months if she's often exposed to secondhand smoke, and another 6 months for any known exposure to lead, arsenic, or mercury. Still too soon? Buy her a gym membership. Life-style factors like exercise, a healthy diet, and low stress will buy you 1 more year of freedom. And don't forget to factor in exactly how many ankle-biters you plan to breed. "If you start thinking about having your first child at 40, you could be in for a lot of difficulty, especially if you plan on having more," says Birrittieri. "You have to plan for your last child, not your first."

**We're hoping my wife will become pregnant. How can I crank up my sperm count naturally?**

It takes more than cojones to get the job done. You need a whole-body approach.

- **Take a multivitamin.** Men with low sperm counts often have deficiencies in zinc, manganese, selenium, and vitamins A, C, and E, says Lani Burkman, PhD, assistant professor of gynecology, obstetrics, and urology at the University at Buffalo (SUNY).
- **Don't take testosterone.** Your T must come from your testicles, says *Men's Health* urology advisor Larry Lipshultz, MD. "If you take testosterone, you're shutting down your own production."
- **Lose weight.** "Fatty tissue converts testosterone to estrogen," says Dr. Lipshultz. No testosterone, no sperm. Regular exercise will help reverse that and can also help you...
- **Cut stress.** Stressful living affects sperm quality, says Dr. Burkman. So work less, sleep more, and pick up a relaxing hobby. Like, say, sex.
- **Stop smoking.** Your sperm confuses nicotine with a natural chemical and overdoses on it, says Dr. Burkman. This can lower sperm count and quality, and can damage its DNA.
- **Consider supplements.** A few new products, such as Fertile One, Proceed, and Fertility Blend, promise help, but there's no scientific proof behind them, says Dr. Lipshultz. They won't hurt you, he says, and may improve quality but not quantity.

### I've been using Propecia and want to have kids. Will it affect my fertility?

Most likely not. Propecia, or finasteride, does have a potentially negative effect on male fertility, but only when sperm production is already borderline.

### How do I discipline my child in public?

Two things are at stake: how you handle the child and how onlookers perceive your handling of the child. Stay cool (a steely calm is good); nobody wants to see two red-faced screamers. If it's a kid-friendly place (zoo, playground), relax in the knowledge that the other parents know it's not your fault. But in an adult setting (bistro, museum), take action. If your charm fails, quickly move the drama out of the main arena. You'll limit your embarrassment and quell the ire of the adults around you.

### How can I connect better with kids?

Loosen up; they're kids, not rattlesnakes. Show emotion and engage the children, whether they're 6 or 16, says Ken Canfield, PhD, founder and president of the National Center for Fathering. With a younger child, get down to his or her eye level to make the conversation more personal. Offer to shake his hand

## PERCENTAGE CHANCE THAT CHILDREN OF OVERWEIGHT PARENTS WILL GROW UP TO BE JUST AS HEAVY: 48

or have him slap you five. Speak to her in a calm, normal tone of voice (no baby talk) and ask open-ended questions. "Tell me about your best friend at school" or "What kind of music do you like to listen to?" lets kids know you're actually interested. Look for common points of connection between you and them and offer anecdotes from personal experience. Avoid the clichéd, tough-guy "When I was your age . . ." and try telling an embarrassing story instead. "Be wise to the power of self-deprecating humor," says Dr. Canfield. "When you can demonstrate some vulnerability, children are willing to listen."

### I got divorced a few years back and am getting remarried in 6 months. How do I break the news to my kids?

"Telling your kids that you're getting remarried is one of the most difficult sales you'll ever have to make," says Jeanette Lofas, PhD, president of the Stepfamily Foundation (www.stepfamily.org). How well it goes depends largely on the relationship they have with your fiancée. "The best way to broach the subject is to do it in a quiet restaurant with a private booth—never at home. This will allow you to talk openly in a setting that's free of distractions and negative associations," says Dr. Lofas. Your fiancée should not be present, as you want to reinforce the idea that the kids' opinions count and that you're not abandoning them. If you get a positive response, ask them to participate in the wedding. This will help them feel like a part of the new union. What-ever happens, though, remember that there are many more conversations like this ahead, so don't go into a lot of detail. Introduce the idea, listen to their concerns, and leave the door open to questions. And remember, your kids do not have veto power.

### My 14-year-old son doesn't talk at all. How do I tell if he's depressed or just being a teenager?

"It's normal for boys to become a little more private once they reach adoles-cence," says David Bennett, PhD, assistant professor of child and adolescent psychiatry at Drexel University in Philadelphia. "However, if you think your son has depression, there are other symptoms to watch for, like changes in appetite, mood, or sleep, or decreased interest in activities he used to enjoy." Depression is a leading cause of adolescent suicide, accounting for roughly 2,000 teen deaths each year in the United States. We don't mean to alarm you, but err on the side of caution. Set aside some time to talk with him one-on-one, coupling it with an activity he enjoys, such as playing catch or fishing. Express your concern, and ask him open-ended questions about what's on his mind. If he doesn't open up, contact his teachers to find out if they've noticed a change in him at school. "It's a delicate situation because your son doesn't want you prying into his affairs, but you have to let him know that you care," says Dr. Bennett.

### Should I get my kid a cell phone?

Is your kid old enough to spend a good deal of time outside your supervision? Is your life full of soccer practices, schedule changes, and late meetings? If so, it may be time to pony up for the family plan.

Think of a cell phone as a safety net. "Practically speaking, if the child is going out on her own, don't you want her to have a way to contact you?" says Paul Saffo, director of the Institute for the Future, a nonprofit technology-research group.

Until your child is old enough to be out of your sight for prolonged periods, teach her how to use your cell in an emergency. For older kids, most phone providers sell password-protected phones to control outgoing calls so you can ensure the phone is used mostly for safety, rather than social reasons.

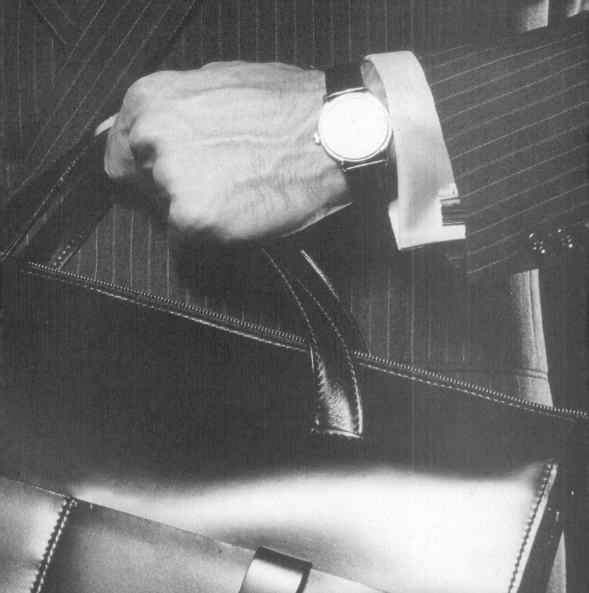

# SEVEN

# WORK SMARTER

# READ UP ON IT

## Money for Everything

Nine simple ways to build seven figures

### by Anya Kamenetz

Finance gurus annoy us. Forgo your daily latte, they tell us, and that $4 a day, compounded over 20 years at 8 percent interest, will grow into $70,000. Fine, but what about this: You like latte. If you were to apply their advice to every aspect of your life, you'd live at the Y, hitchhike to work, and eat three squares of wheat bread a day. And forget sex: Each 12-pack of Trojans you buy now would be worth $173 at retirement.

Our point: Their advice may help you save, but it won't help you live. And besides, it's not necessary. Retiring rich isn't that difficult. You simply need to recognize your spending strengths and weaknesses and learn how to exploit the former while suppressing the latter.

And, actually, you don't even need to worry about the learning part because we have your lessons right here. We polled 1,600 visitors to www.menshealth. com about their spending habits and financial priorities. Then we asked a handful of money experts across the country for their best no-hassle tips—simple ways to save more without denying yourself the things that make life worth living. Their advice is universal, but how you execute it depends on the type of spender you are. To figure that out, take this one-question self-test.

Think, don't look:

How much cash do you have in your wallet right now?

A. Could be $100, could be $3. I don't really know.
B. $200 or more in crisp, new 20s and 50s.
C. One emergency 20, folded up and stuck in the credit-card slot.

If you answered A, you're a Sleepwalker. You spend on impulse for big and small stuff alike, never thinking about your budget. At the end of the month, you wonder where it all went. Everyone has a little bit of Sleepwalker in him— that's why crafty marketing experts put candy bars and *Us Weekly* magazine at the checkout counter. But a bad case of Sleepwalker can mean overdue bills and falling short of long-term financial goals without even realizing it.

If you answered B, you're a Status Spender. You may be in a commission-based profession like real estate, sales, or finance. Regardless, you're living large and want friends, colleagues, and ladies to know it—new cars, expensive dinners, the latest tech gear. The danger, of course, comes when your lifestyle inevitably outruns your paycheck.

If you answered C, you're a Scrimper, with a tight lock on your finances. You probably think you don't need our advice, but scrimping has two major downsides. First, you could be denying yourself the pleasures of a job well done, which sets you up for occasional binge spending. Second, you may not be able to part with a large chunk of change, even when it's a wise investment.

Okay, now that you know yourself, here's what to do.

## 1. CREATE A PERSONAL EXPENSE ACCOUNT

Seventy percent of you have a savings account, but less than half of you use it. This wouldn't be a criminal offense, except that almost 30 percent of you regularly pay overdraft or late fees because you don't have enough money in your account to pay your bills on time, every time. The solution: Open a checking account just for household expenses with whatever's required to avoid monthly service fees (around $2,000, typically). Next, figure out roughly how much your monthly expenses—everything from electricity to entertainment—should run, and direct-deposit that much into the account from your paycheck. Put the rest of your paycheck into your savings account and let it accumulate until you need it (we'll talk about that in #9, on page 242). Not only have you just taken the guesswork out of saving, you've also created a budget without the hassle of doing a monthly line-by-line accounting of what you've spent. If you have $2,100 left in your checking account at the end of 1 month, spend the extra $100 the next. If you have $1,900 left, cut back on expenses the following month.

**Sleepwalkers.** Pay your bills online. It's quicker, and you can set up automatic payments for all recurring expenses. "Often, [Sleepwalkers] aren't late

THE AVERAGE GUY'S ANNUAL INCOME:
# $39,429

because they don't have the money," says Judy Lawrence, financial counselor in Cupertino, California, and author of *The Budget Kit*. "They just don't make the time."

**Status Spenders.** Forget online banking and take the time to balance your checkbook the old-fashioned way. It'll make you more aware of what you're spending each month.

**Scrimpers.** You're going to be tempted to start building a balance in your checking account. Resist. "You've set your budget, and you know how much is okay to spend," says Lawrence. So spend it.

## 2. GO TO THE ATM ONCE A WEEK, NO MORE

Thirty percent of you say you make most everyday purchases with cash, while 50 percent of you use a debit card. Some financial experts favor cash, others prefer plastic, but all agree that visiting the ATM more than once a week is a red flag. This takes some planning and discipline. "If I have $40 in my wallet," says Mike Furois, a certified financial planner in Phoenix, "it's easy to spend $35 in 2 days and hang on to the other $5 for a week."

**Sleepwalkers.** Limiting ATM visits is especially important for you. Take out the same amount each week—preferably no more than $100—and force yourself to make it last.

**Status Spenders.** Don't carry more than $200 at a time. "Some of my clients never have less than $500 in their wallets," Furois says. "I try to get them to cut back gradually, so they don't blow hundreds of dollars at once."

**Scrimpers.** Split your weekly withdrawal into envelopes marked "groceries," "gas," and so on. If you have any left come Saturday, go out for a guilt-free dinner or movie.

## 3. TAKE A SALARY CUT

Two-thirds of you have a 401(k), 403(b), or IRA account, but only 20 percent of you are putting 10 percent or more of your paychecks toward retirement. More disturbing, 21 percent of you aren't saving for retirement at all. "Our younger clients not only are not maxing out their 401(k)s," says Scott Kahan, a certified financial planner in New York City, "but they're not taking advantage of their employers' matching funds—that's free money." The tax benefits amount to free money as well: Every $1,000 you contribute saves $300 in taxes. Our experts agree: Don't put less than 10 percent of your salary into your retirement plan each month. Because of the tax benefits, your take-home pay will drop by only 7 percent. That seems like a lot, but trust us, you'll never miss it. And in 10 years, you'll be giddy every time your 401(k) statement arrives. Oh, if you're under 30, put all your money in stocks. At 30, start drizzling in cash, bonds, and other safe investments.

**Sleepwalkers.** You can't be trusted to make your own retirement contributions, so set up automatic payments.

**Status Spenders.** Don't you dare buy that boat until you've maxed your contributions to your 401(k) and Roth IRA. Don't have a Roth? Put down this book and open one now.

**Scrimpers.** If rolling the dice with stocks has you hyperventilating, go with a balanced fund—a preset mix of stocks, bonds, and cash. It won't appreciate as fast, but you'll be able to sleep at night.

## 4. POSTPONE GADGET PURCHASES FOR 3 MONTHS

The electronics store is the place guys are most likely to spend more than they intend, according to 59 percent of you. In fact, almost half of you say that if your TV broke next week, you'd instantly replace it with a $1,500 or even $5,000 flat-screen or plasma version. That's a lot of money to spend hastily. Hence, our 3-month moratorium.

# WHAT TO BUY WHEN
### Turns out, you can time the market

### New Car

**When:** Last week of December
**Why:** Dealers are scrambling to hit monthly and annual quotas, says Phil Reed, of Edmunds.com. And don't buy the current year's model—it's already depreciated an average of 14 percent.

### Cruise

**When:** April or November
**Why:** That's when cruise lines reposition their ships for seasonal route changes. "You'll save 50 percent or more," says Bill Miller, author of more than 60 books about the cruise industry.

### Yellowstone Vacation

**When:** May
**Why:** Most of the snow has melted by then, so almost everything is open, the weather is usually pleasant, and the park averages only a third as many visitors as it does in July.

**Sleepwalkers.** Don't even walk into Best Buy until you've decided what you want and it's time to make your purchase. Lawrence knows your type. "One of my clients, a guy in his 20s, goes into the electronics store to comparison shop. But once he's there, he can't help himself and spends far more than he can afford."

**Status Spenders.** Use the time to do background research, compare features, and, most important, save enough to pay in cash. If your friends ask about the delay, tell them you're just waiting for the next iProduct.

**Scrimpers.** Save a little extra so you can purchase a better-quality product. It'll last longer and work better than that cheap knockoff you've been eyeing.

## 5. SEND AN EXTRA $10 TO YOUR FRIENDS AT MASTERCARD

Just over half of you confess to carrying a credit-card balance, and one in five owes more than a month's salary and makes the minimum payments. Credit-card debt, we don't need to tell you, is financial suicide. "If you add just $10 to your minimum payment," says Lawrence, "you'll save thousands in the long run." Example: Say you owe $5,000 at 21 percent interest. Paying

## Mutual Funds

**When:** Early in the year

**Why:** You won't be taxed on money that hasn't yet grown, says Jason Zweig, a columnist at *Money* magazine. Buy on December 31, say, and you'll receive end-of-year dividends—and a tax bill.

## Outdoor Gear

**When:** 2 to 3 months before the season

**Why:** You'll save up to 20 percent by scooping up last year's equipment, says Kristin Hostetter, gear editor at *Backpacker* magazine. "If it was great gear last year, it'll be great gear this year."

## Furniture

**When:** October or April

**Why:** Stores are unloading last season's pieces, says Kenneth Brown, host of HGTV's *reDesign*. "These are sample sales, so the pieces may be dinged. But you'll save 50 to 60 percent."

$100 a month, it'll take almost 10 years to satisfy the debt. Pay $110 a month, though, and you'll finish 2½ years earlier.

**Sleepwalkers.** Seven percent of our survey respondents have no idea how much credit-card debt they have. That's quintessential Sleepwalker. Most credit cards let you set up automatic monthly payments. Do so.

**Status Spenders.** If your income depends heavily on commissions or bonuses, you're most at risk of outsize (five-figure) credit-card debt that accumulates quietly when money flow is low. Avoid it by putting only purchases of more than $1,000 on your credit card. Since we told you not to withdraw more than $200 at a time, other purchases will require a special trip to the ATM, giving you time to reconsider.

**Scrimpers.** Credit-card debt drives you crazy—so crazy, in fact, that you often contemplate cutting up your cards. Don't. You need them for emergencies and to maintain a good credit rating. Just go with your strength: Systematically chip away at your debt, and it'll be gone in no time.

## 6. BUY ONLY ONE ROUND A NIGHT, PREFERABLY THE LAST ONE

Walk into a restaurant or bar and your cash does an impressive disappearing act: 28 percent of you admit that your wallet comes out most freely when you're among friends, 85 percent say you splurge "often" for dinner, and 60 percent tell us you regularly purchase premium beer. "Men, especially single men, feel pressure when they're going out with friends or co-workers: 'I'll pick up the tab, don't worry about it.' It's an ego thing," says Kahan. Go ahead, pick up a round, but wait until later in the night, when your buds aren't so thirsty for suds.

**Sleepwalkers.** Leave your credit cards at home, lest you be tempted to put the whole night on your Visa.

**Status Spenders.** Develop a taste for quality scotch—one glass is perfect for sipping and far cheaper than three premium beers. Plus, you'll look sophisticated.

**Scrimpers.** Steer the gathering to "a great dive bar near the office." As long as the place is sufficiently grungy, no one will suspect your real motivation: to hold down costs.

## 7. MAKE EVERY THIRD DATE CHEAP, FREE, OR DUTCH

Ah, romance. You can't put a price on it, but it costs you dearly. Seventy-seven percent of you say you almost always pay, with half of you typically dropping $150 or more on a big date. Seven percent say it's not unusual to spend $500 if you're really into her. We're not suggesting you become miserly, just that you mix it up. A run in the park can end happily, too.

**Sleepwalkers.** Set up a regular, low-cost date with your girl: coffee and the paper at her place on Sundays, perhaps.

**Status Spenders.** Swear off gifts and expensive dates ($200 or more) for the first 3 months of any new relationship, or at least until you know you're serious about her, recommends Dean Harman, a certified financial planner in The Woodlands, Texas.

**Scrimpers.** Both working late? Take her out for dessert (not dinner) at a nice restaurant afterward. She'll think it's neat, not cheap.

## 8. SPLURGE ON SHOES, NOT SHIRTS

The most expensive items in your closet should be the most durable, says Harman. Many of you have this principle down: 35 percent say you're more likely to splurge on shoes than on shirts or suits. In fact, nearly half of you say your nicest dress shirt cost only $40.

**Sleepwalkers.** Reorganize your closet. If you know exactly what you

# INVESTMENTS IN GOOD LIVING
### Because some things are never a waste of money

**$5 mustard.** Sure, Gulden's will do just fine. But add the right spicy, grainy mustard and a hot dog becomes a different animal. A hot jackal, perhaps.

**$1,800 business-class seat.** Once a year, be a really high roller. Your destination, no matter how bland, will suddenly seem like Monte Carlo.

**$30 case of beer.** Bell's Two Hearted Ale. Fuller's ESB. Victory Prima Pils. If you're going to molest your liver, do it with class.

**$200 spa gift certificate.** Not for you. For her. A man with a pampered woman watches more ball games without interruption.

**$18 monthly HDTV package.** The clarity is so cool you might forget that your cable company is completely ripping you off.

**$1,500 set of irons.** Buying new clubs more than three times in a lifetime is a duffer's play. Regrip them often and pass them to your son when he breaks 100.

**$500 pair of concert tickets.** Pick one must-see event every year. Forget the cash. Remember the set list.

**$30 concert shirt.** Pick one at that very show, in fact. In 10 years you'll have a genuine vintage T-shirt for any cool-casual occasion.

**$30,000 (or more!) vehicle.** No, not a mommy van. Imagine: a vehicle you'll still love to drive after 6 years. Imagine: a vehicle still worth something after 6 years. Life's way too short for a substandard ride.

have—what still fits, what still looks new—you'll be less likely to buy on impulse.

**Status Spenders.** Fine, buy premium brands, but only when they're on sale. Even Neiman Marcus has outlet stores.

**Scrimpers.** When it comes to clothes, spend 20 percent more per item than you plan to. You'll get better quality, and you'll stand a little taller.

## 9. KEEP THE BIG PRIZE IN SIGHT

What are you saving for? A house? A car? A dream vacation? Early retirement? "Figure out how you want to reward yourself in the future," says Kahan. "Then work backward. How will you get there?"

**Sleepwalkers.** Pick a 5-year goal—far enough out to force you to think beyond the short term but not so far that you'll forget about it by next month. Next, create annual yardsticks with which to measure success. To strengthen your resolve, make a small investment this year. Saving for a motorcycle? Buy a helmet and take lessons.

**Status Spenders.** Set a 20-year goal. Why? "One year you might make $150,000," says Furois, "and you think you'll always have that kind of money." Setting a long-term goal, one that you can achieve whether you make $75,000 or $150,000, will keep you focused on building wealth.

**Scrimpers.** Reward your discipline. Even if you already have a long-term goal, give back to yourself each year—if not a vacation, then something useful, like a new lawn mower. Or, even better, a lawn-mowing service. Irresponsible? Maybe, but you deserve it.

# Good Buddies, Bad Business

Always dreamed of going into business with a close pal? A few lessons from reformed optimists who lost their money—and their friendships

**by George Mannes**

In high school, you dreamed of forming a rock band with your best friend. Now that the two of you are older, the fantasy has morphed into creating the next Google. But just as becoming the Plant and Page of Central High brought on its share of beefs ("'Stairway to Heaven' follows 'Moby Dick' on the set list, man!"), the path to becoming the next Sergey Brin and Larry Page is also fraught with heated head-banging. So how do you get from the garage to a billion-dollar intellectual property owner (IPO) without wrecking the friendship (or yourself) in the process?

The major problem is that the same personality traits that make a loyal companion may not be the best qualities for a business partner. "Friends who go into business together are often not very clear with each other about what their expectations are," says Susan Lazar, a Minneapolis-based consultant who works with closely held and family-owned businesses to create clarity in communications, planning, leadership, and resource management.

Anyone looking for a case that illustrates Lazar's point need look no further than Hollywood agent Michael Ovitz and Walt Disney CEO Michael Eisner. For years, they were close friends. But that was before the two of them agreed in 1995 that Ovitz should join Disney as president—a 14-month tenure that proved unsatisfactory for Disney and disastrous for the friendship. Upon Ovitz's departure in December 1996, Eisner wrote in a memo, "He is a psychopath (doesn't know right from wrong), cannot tell the truth."

In a Delaware courtroom last fall, at a trial devoted to his unhappy presidency, Ovitz marveled at how a friend of 25 years could turn on him in 60 days: "I live to this day with a 25-year hole in my life."

According to attorneys, organizational consultants, and veterans of successful start-up companies, these disasters can be avoided—if friends are willing to sit down before they sign a partnership agreement and talk through

**PERCENTAGE OF MEN WHO ARE UNHAPPY WITH THE SIZE OF THEIR PAYCHECKS: 49**

how they'll feel and react at hypothetical moments. They need to perform emotional due diligence and blue-sky tough questions: Who will have the final say on key decisions? How many hours are in a perfect workweek?

It's always easier for partners to tackle these issues before a business is operational. Otherwise, Lazar says, "habits are already established, patterns are already set, and they have to backtrack." To avoid slipping into bad habits, follow these six rules.

## DOUBLE-TEAM IN THE NBA—NOT IN A START-UP

A major issue to settle before launching a business is who will be responsible for what. Even if your skills are similar, it's wasted effort—and a cause of friction—to double-team responsibilities. Instead, divide management geographically, the way Andy Pickup and Rikki Tahta did after they founded Ark Information Services, a distributor of investment research, in 1989.

The two Englishmen met as MBA students at Columbia University in the 1980s. Both had strong backgrounds in finance, marketing, and operations, so they moved to different continents: One ran the U.S. operation from New York and the other ran the European side of the business from London. They swapped apartments and offices every few months.

"You have to give each other space, trust each other 100 percent, value the friendship over the activity, and respect the other person's differential skills," says Pickup of their division of labor. "If you can't check those off, you have a problem."

## WATCH OUT FOR YOKO SYNDROME

Of course, business partners need to trust each other. But it doesn't stop there. They need to earn the faith of their partner's partner—his or her spouse. Why? Two words: Yoko Ono. When someone is forced to choose sides between his spouse and a business partner, it's the business partner who walks the long and winding road.

"There's a lot of pillow talk," says Norm Stoehr, founder of Inner Circle International, a roundtable for entrepreneurs. "I wouldn't go into business with someone anymore unless I knew his spouse was in agreement with our collaborative vision."

## DECIDE ON A CAPTAIN KIRK

Setting up a 50-50 partnership is "one of the most lethal decisions two partners can make," says Don Taylor, executive director of a business incubator network based at West Texas A&M University. "Someone has to be 51 percent and someone has to be 49 percent when it comes to decision making." Ensemble Beverage, a Montgomery, Alabama, company, is a good case study for the type of unforeseen issues that can arise when a leadership structure isn't hammered out in advance.

After he got laid off in 2001 from a job with Coca-Cola, James Harris sought solace during a regular night out with local alumni of his old fraternity. He had already told his Omega Psi Phi brothers about an idea he had to sell Southern-style juices; that night the guys told him it was time to launch the business. "After my fifth shot of tequila, I said, 'You know what? We can do it.'"

Bit by bit, those fraternity brothers joined the venture. Nathan Shaw ponied up money for a big stake in the company and later worked full-time after leaving his pharmaceutical-sales job. Robert Smith came on full-time after working on a losing political campaign in 2002. T. D. Chism, an army officer then stationed in Montgomery, helped out part-time and later became a partner.

When Ensemble started out, the partners mixed batches of lemonade in Harris's backyard. Now they've outsourced manufacturing and are selling 700 cases a month, up from 300 in 2003. But they're still not profitable, and they've had their share of conflicts, like the blowup in November 2003, when Harris and Shaw spent 3 hours arguing in an Auburn University parking lot. Shaw was unhappy that Harris wasn't sharing information about pending deals and that he wasn't yielding any authority. "He really wanted to run the company as a sole proprietorship," says Shaw. "I said, 'You should have told me that a long, long time ago.'"

## CREATE A CONFLICT-RESOLUTION STRUCTURE

If you still choose to run your company as a copresidency, then you need to have a prearranged mechanism for settling disputes, such as an advisory board or paid arbiter.

Jay Marks and Jon Katz, who practice law in Silver Spring, Maryland, employ a less-formal variation of this. It's what they call the 24-Hour Rule. "We just embargo whatever it is that's really pissing us off for 24 hours," says Marks, whose disagreements with Katz date back to elementary-school days.

So 2 years ago, when Marks, without consulting Katz, awarded a raise to a legal secretary whose job performance Katz thought was unsatisfactory, they invoked the rule. "I realized I shouldn't be doing things like that without consulting my law partner," says Marks. "He realized that in the grand scheme of things it wasn't such a big deal."

## HAVE AN EXIT PLAN

What partners need, says Dennis Murrell, an attorney in Louisville, Kentucky, is the equivalent of a prenuptial agreement, to spell out who gets what after the breakup and who owes what to whom.

Assuming it's a 50-50 partnership, says Murrell, partners should set it up so that if it's time to part company, one owner sets a price for half the company and the other owner decides if he's a buyer or seller at that price. Or the two can leave the valuation to a mediator or professional appraiser.

## KILL THE FRIENDSHIP TO SAVE THE BUSINESS

That's one lesson Jim Volz and Barbara Carlyle learned when they teamed with a financial backer to start a San Jose, California, business-furniture dealership out of Carlyle's family room.

Though Volz and Carlyle were never romantically involved, they were close enough friends to go camping together. Volz was "Uncle Jimmy" to Carlyle's kids. Friendship and business went smoothly for the first few years, but both turned ugly during Silicon Valley's early 1990s downturn. "It got to the point where we weren't even talking to each other," says Volz.

As a last-ditch effort to save the company, they brought in Rick Eigenbrod, PhD, an organizational psychologist and a consultant to business owners.

Eigenbrod helped Volz see what strengths Carlyle brought to the business and why he wanted to partner with her in the first place, recalls Volz. Their business, now known as Pivot Interiors, recovered, but their friendship clearly suffered. "I had to make the hard decision that we couldn't stay friends and socialize if our business was to thrive," says Carlyle. "It was like [we had] too much of each other."

It's a bittersweet ending, and one that illustrates the value (and fragility) of friendship. "Friendship itself can really become a business asset," says Eigenbrod. But like so many other assets, it may need to be liquidated to keep the business afloat.

# Creativity Unleashed

Make the right impression and land the business with these steps
from one of the ad game's best

**interview by Matt Bean**

Think big. Wieden + Kennedy, the ad agency that brought you Air Jordan, the Miller High Life man, and those wacky SportsCenter commercials, has been elevating clients to pop-culture-icon status for 23 years. Behind many of these successful campaigns are creative director Jelly Helm and W12, the in-house ad school at W+K's home office in Portland, Oregon.

**Act stupid.** "Our philosophy is to come in ignorant every day. The idea of retaining ignorance is sort of counterintuitive, but it subverts a lot of [problems] that come from absolute mastery. If you think you know the answer better than somebody else does, you become closed to being fresh," Helm says.

**Shut up.** "The first thing we do when we meet with clients is listen. We try to figure out what their problems are. Then we come back with questions, not solutions. We write these out and put them on the wall. And then we circle the ones that we think are interesting. More often than not, the questions hold the answer."

**Always say yes.** "What I've learned from improvisation is to let go of outcome and just say yes to whatever the situation is. If you say an idea is bad, you're creating conflict—you're breaking an improv rule. You want an energy flow that moves you forward, as opposed to a creative stasis."

**Chase talent.** "Find people who make you better. It's best to be the least talented person in the room. It's reciprocal. It challenges you to keep up."

**Be fearless.** "Do anything, say anything. In the words of our president, Dan Wieden, 'You're not useful to me until you've made three momentous mistakes.' He knows that if you try not to make mistakes, you miss out on the value of learning from them."

# SCI-GUY

## Take a Break

The Man isn't keeping you down, at least in terms of total poundage. Regularly working overtime may inflate your weight, according to University of Helsinki researchers. The scientists tracked the work habits and weights of nearly 1,800 men over a 12-month period and found that those who regularly logged late hours were 36 percent more likely to tip the scales at above-normal weights than the 9-to-5ers. And too much takeout may not be the only culprit, says study author Tea Lallukka, MSc. The stress of a string of 12-hour days can cause a spike in cortisol, a hormone that stimulates hunger. If you can't keep to a 40-hour week, make sure you don't skip exercise. It burns calories and releases endorphins, a natural antidote to excess cortisol.

Another study found that it's no wonder it feels as if the boss is always on your back. Logging overtime increases a man's risk of back pain, according to a recent University of Massachusetts study. Information gathered from nearly 11,000 employees revealed that men who worked overtime had a 61 percent higher risk of an on-the-job injury than those who punched out after 8 straight, with back pain topping the list of complaints. What's more, white-collar workers suffered just as many injuries as their blue-collar brethren, says lead author Allard Dembe, ScD. "Working long hours may induce stress and fatigue," he explains, which can cause a person to forget to stand up and stretch. Try to grab a 15-minute nap twice per shift.

## Use Your Sick Days

A new study reveals that men who refuse to stay home from work when they have a cold, the flu, or another illness may sabotage their heart health. British researchers reviewed the health records and work attendance of 5,071 men over a period of 3 years and discovered that men who punched in despite feeling ill had double the risk of serious heart problems of those who called in sick. The mental stress of working while feeling lousy may increase the odds of an artery-clogging event, says Mika Kivimaki, PhD, the lead study author. Or it may be that the same men who ignore minor illnesses are more likely to ignore symptoms of heart disease. Whatever the reason, there's more to be gained from quarantining yourself at home—faster recovery, no chance of infecting co-workers, less risk of heart trouble—than by playing the part of company martyr.

## Wake Up

Falling down on the job? Falling down tired? You may have sleep apnea—or more likely something masquerading as the condition. Daytime sleepiness is an often-overlooked sign of diabetes or depression, according to a new Pennsylvania State University study. Researchers surveyed 1,741 people about their energy levels, then monitored them in a sleep lab overnight. Depression was the most common culprit, followed by excess weight, diabetes, and, in last place, sleep apnea. A misdiagnosis could mean ineffective treatment, so go for a sleep study if you're experiencing daytime drowsiness, says lead author Edward Bixler, PhD.

## Put Out the Fire

You're not lazy; you might just have acid reflux. Heartburn can make a person less productive at work, according to a new study in the *American Journal of Gastroenterology*. A study of 642 patients with acid reflux revealed that sufferers lose an average of 16 hours of productive work time per week, most likely as a result of sleep disturbances caused by heartburn. When the patients took 40 milligrams of the acid suppressor Nexium (esomeprazole magnesium), their productivity increased by 72 percent. "Many people don't realize that their heartburn—particularly if it occurs at night—can really affect their performance at work," says William Orr, PhD, the study's lead author. If you think acid reflux may be turning you into a slacker and you've already tried over-the-counter remedies, ask your doctor for a prescription proton-pump inhibitor.

**AVERAGE NUMBER OF MINUTES A MAN SPENDS SITTING DOWN DURING A TYPICAL WORKDAY: 209**

# Tell the One About…

Opening your next meeting with the joke about the cheerleader and the ball boy is not a good idea. But a new University of Washington at Bothell study suggests that in certain kinds of workplaces, sexual banter can promote camaraderie and bonding among co-workers. Such interaction can "make people feel happy, free, and more human," says Kari Lerum, PhD, and that may lead to greater efficiency. Lerum stresses that her findings are specific to the service industry (she collected her data in restaurants) and apply only where employees are fairly equal in status and work closely together. She adds, "It only works if everyone is on board."

# Ignore the Heels

When does a hot woman turn a man cold? When she's his boss. Men and women react negatively toward female managers who dress provocatively, according to a new study published in the journal *Psychology of Women Quarterly*. A boss in sexy clothes tended to prompt feelings of irritation and frustration in study participants, who viewed her as less competent and intelligent than a female boss in conservative clothing. The data show that the negative reaction applied only to women in high-status positions. Men and women "do not like it if they think a woman is using sexiness manipulatively, to create an unfair advantage," says study author Peter Glick, PhD, professor of psychology at Lawrence University. Never mind the clothes, Glick says, and "try to judge her by how well she does her job."

# Talk It Out

Trouble at home doesn't always stay at home. People in bad marriages are more than twice as likely to report stress at work as those who are happily wed, according to a British study. Unhappy spouses also have higher diastolic blood pressures. "You might not be conscious of it, but you take [marriage problems] with you to work," says study author Rosalind Barnett, PhD. "Talk seriously with your partner and try to work things out, because it can affect your health." A separate study in *Psychosomatic Medicine* shows that having a supportive partner decreases stress. After positive contact with their spouses, men showed increases in their levels of oxytocin, a hormone that reduces the production of stress hormones and protects the heart.

## Shrink Your Workload

Don't chain yourself to your desk. In a recent Australian study of 1,579 people, researchers discovered that workers whose jobs require more than 6 hours of chair time a day are up to 68 percent more likely to wind up overweight or obese than those who sit less. When the scientists analyzed the data by gender, they found that total sitting time was associated with a body-mass index (BMI) of over 25 in men, but not in women. The likely reason: On average, the women sat for 20 minutes less a day than the men, says lead researcher Kerry Mummery, PhD. To make sure the Man isn't keeping you down all day long, use a stopwatch to track your occupational sitting time. Take the average of 3 days' readings, then make a conscious effort to cut 20 minutes off that number by handling office communications in person instead of by phone or e-mail or by going for a walk during your lunch break.

## Speak Up

British civil servants in low-ranking jobs are three times more likely to develop type-2 diabetes than those with higher-level positions, according to a study published in the *Archives of Internal Medicine*. Workers who felt that they weren't being fairly compensated for their efforts were at the greatest risk of developing diabetes.

# WHAT'S NEW

## Sweat-Less Shoes

No-sweat dress shoes might sound like something you'd see on an infomercial at 3:00 a.m., but they will leave your feet dry as long as the insoles of the shoes, such as those from Ecco, have various-size micropores that allow vapor to pass through. Beware of shoes that claim to wick away sweat by using waterproof material like Gore-Tex fabrics. These shoes failed hundreds of Michigan State University thermal tests of lining variations, and testers found no difference in foot temperature or antiperspiration, says Ray Fredericksen, MS, of Sport Biomechanics. "Unless the shoe design incorporates a ventilation system, such as an open mesh panel, they will not breathe well and let perspiration out."

## Speedy Smart Phone

Wi-Fi and 3G network support make the Nokia E61 a fast, flexible unit. You can even make Internet phone calls. Downside: no camera ($400–$500, www. nokia.com).

## Red-Hot Sack

Some briefcase haters argue that alpha boys just bring their brains with them. We love this arrogance, but it's a relic of pre-laptop antiquity. Rule: Carry as little luggage as possible. If you have to schlep only a subpoena or two, a sleek leather briefcase makes a polished presentation. But when you have your computer, the Coach Legacy Leather Map Bag, a lightweight, tanned leather messenger bag, is a great choice. But no stuffing it. Nobody should think

**PERCENTAGE OF WORKING AMERICANS WHO SAY THEY ROUTINELY EAT LUNCH AT THEIR DESKS: 35**

you've jammed a change of undies and a sandwich in there (www.coach. com).

## Blend-N-Go Cup

Mix up your morning carpool smoothie right in the travel cup with Oster's Blend-N-Go cup and almost any Oster blender base. Churn up your ingredients, flip the cup, replace the blade with the travel lid, and head out the door. Seconds later you're behind the wheel, on time and ready for your first slurp.

## Quick Brew

You love strong coffee; she insists on tea. You can both get your caffeine fix. The Krups Home Café pod brewing machine brews both coffee and tea simultaneously in 1 minute (about $120, www.krups.com).

# T A K E 5

## Check Out

Five mental vacations that let you bounce back better than before

**A** week at Sandals may recharge you physically, but you'll probably arrive home even more mentally exhausted than before you left. Here's how to give your mind some well-deserved R&R.

**If you have 5 minutes.** Try the gravity-free workout. Eyes open or closed, visualize your body taking up a larger and larger space, until it seems to float away. It'll feel as if you're in a hot-air balloon, without the view.

**If you have 10 minutes.** Think of nothing. This is hard at first. Our trick: Think of a nonsense syllable (like "smo") over and over again, and let nothing else enter your mind. Try this, and after 10 minutes, you'll feel refreshed.

**If you have 3 hours.** Play hooky, using technology. Let the sheer depth of the Internet carry you away—news, music, women, ancient Icelandic customs, whatever. The goal is to enter a world outside yourself so you can mentally shut down.

**If you have 3 days.** OD on forbidden fruit. That is, saturate your life with something you truly love. It could be 1960s cartoons or skinny women or Fox News. Doesn't matter, as long as it's legal. You'll feel reinvigorated and ready to return to the real world.

**If you have a week.** Change your sleep patterns. Instead of sleeping 8 hours at night, nap for 4 hours twice a day—from 4:00 to 8:00 p.m. and 4:00 to 8:00 a.m. The day will feel twice as long, as if you are taking a 2-week vacation.

# MEN'S HEALTH
## QUIZ

## Should You Quit Your Job?

Take our test before you tell your boss to pound sand.

**1. Which important occasion did you miss?**
   A. My fraternity reunion
   B. A crucial board meeting
   C. My kid's softball championship game

Missing special family events means it's time to reassess, says Ronald Downey, PhD, professor of industrial and organizational psychology at Kansas State University. "Many people are making decisions to downsize their jobs to accommodate their families," he says. Look first at your time-sucking commute; see if you can do more work at home.

**2. What's keeping you at your job?**
   A. This gig is part of my long-term plan.
   B. It's all I'm qualified to do.
   C. I don't want to move.

Unhappy employees who think they have to stay put just become more miserable, says Arthur Brief, PhD, professor at the Freeman School of Business at Tulane University. Many "fail to search for alternatives because they think they're unmarketable," Dr. Brief says. If that sounds like you, start reading want ads and call a headhunter to see what the truth is.

**3. How do you keep in touch off-site?**
   A. I'm a crackberry addict
   B. My cell phone and mobile e-mail
   C. Maybe my cell, if I decide to turn it on

If you're never off the job, it might be time to get a new one. "Somewhere along the way, you lose the time for creative thought," Dr. Downey says. "The quantity [of communication] goes up, but the quality goes down." Try shutting off your BlackBerry in the evening and on weekends. If that doesn't work, consider looking for a job that doesn't require one.

### 4. How does your boss make you feel?
A. Incompetent
B. Overqualified
C. Challenged

The biggest factor in job satisfaction is an employee's relationship with his supervisor, says Dr. Downey. But 52 percent of Americans say their relationship with management is negative. A supervisor "should entrust you with tasks he would have done himself," Dr. Downey says. If you're not getting some hefty assignments, maybe you should look elsewhere.

### 5. You and your co-workers talk about . . .
A. How miserable work is
B. The latest episode of *Lost*
C. Nothing. We don't really talk.

Most people thrive when they have a social network at the office, but not when that network becomes complaint central. "People who are unhappy at their jobs, who bitch and moan to each other, end up making it worse," Dr. Brief says. Keep office talk light, and don't unload all your negativity at home: "It negatively affects those relationships, too."

### 6. How old are you?
A. In my 20s
B. In my 30s
C. In my 40s

It's common for young people to be unhappy at work. If you're older and feeling down, it might be time to move on. "People tend to change careers in their forties and fifties more than at other times," says Bettina Seidman, a New York City career counselor. If you don't find work fulfilling, shop new fields by way of graduate classes and professional associations.

**PERCENTAGE OF PEOPLE WHO HAVE HAD SEX AT WORK: 23**

### 7. You could describe your job in . . .
A. A sentence
B. 30 seconds
C. A 20-minute PowerPoint presentation

Wearing too many hats can destroy your focus and make a happy employee a miserable one. "Role overload becomes role ambiguity, and that becomes really difficult for people," Dr. Downey says. "It leads to even greater stress and anxiety." Sometimes stepping down from a management position can help you rediscover a job you once loved.

### 8. Do you stick to a reliable work schedule?
A. Never
B. Usually, unless a crisis strikes
C. Always

Office disorganization can lead to job burnout. A survey of 1,100 employees in the *Journal of Occupational & Organizational Psychology* found that well-defined procedures, clean and safe work spaces, and clear goals made workers healthier and happier. People in more structured jobs also felt more committed to staying put.

### Scoring

| | | | |
|---|---|---|---|
| 1. | A = 3 | B = 2 | C = 1 |
| 2. | A = 3 | B = 1 | C = 2 |
| 3. | A = 1 | B = 2 | C = 3 |
| 4. | A = 1 | B = 2 | C = 3 |
| 5. | A = 1 | B = 3 | C = 2 |
| 6. | A = 3 | B = 2 | C = 1 |
| 7. | A = 3 | B = 2 | C = 1 |
| 8. | A = 1 | B = 2 | C = 3 |

**18 to 24 points:** We hear the gold watch they hand out is a really nice one.
**11 to 17 points:** Glad you're happy, but keep your eyes open.
**10 points or less:** You still here?

# BURNING QUESTIONS

**I'm drowning in e-mail at the office. How can I get my colleagues to send me less of it?**

"The best way to receive fewer e-mails is to send fewer e-mails," says Kaitlin Duck Sherwood, author of *Overcome Email Overload*. If you're copied on a message from a co-worker, don't respond unless it's vitally important that you do so (being copied generally means that the sender doesn't require a response anyway).

Similarly, when you send an e-mail, blind-copy the bulk of your recipients. This will keep them from replying to anyone but you and from starting up side conversations by making liberal use of the "reply all" button. If no reply is needed to an e-mail you send out, say so in the body of the message. And when making a request, end with "thanks in advance" to avoid the "thanks/you're welcome" loop. Finally, "never include a rhetorical question," says Sherwood. "Inevitably, you'll get answers."

**My company gives raises of only 3 percent, but I deserve 20 percent. How do I get it?**

Tell your boss. He'll give you a raft of horse hockey about how nobody gets more. That's a lie. Not only is he getting more, but he also has access to the corporate jet, a car allowance, and other goodies you can't imagine. What you need to do is make such a total pain in the ass of yourself that it becomes preferable for him to grant you the bigger raise.

Realize that being an annoyance is a delicate game. You have to modulate your act with subtlety and grace and continue to perform your job function with great distinction. Work hard and skillfully, and push, push, push. In the end, you'll get more money than the polite people who listen to the party line and accept their yearly bowlful of gruel.

**One of my co-workers comes into my office all the time to shoot the breeze. How can I politely shut him up?**

Easy: Be honest. "Jerry, I can't talk right now. I'm really under the gun. Another time, maybe." If he keeps popping in, go on the offensive: "I'd love to talk, but I'm slammed. How about I stop by when I'm free?" Then make sure your visit is a quick one.

### How can I tell if my company is tracking my Web surfing?

Unless your computer skills outperform those of your IT department, you can't. But it's safe to assume that you're being watched, tracked, and recorded. A survey by the American Management Association and the ePolicy Institute found that 76 percent of companies monitor employees' Web connections, and 26 percent of those companies had fired employees for "inappropriate" Internet use. What's more, 36 percent of companies surveyed record keystrokes, 50 percent review computer files, and 55 percent retain e-mail.

"There are three big reasons for this surveillance: a growing concern over security breaches, the use of e-mail evidence in workplace lawsuits, and the fear that inappropriate computer use will embarrass the company and lower productivity," explains Nancy Flynn, executive director of the ePolicy Institute.

Such monitoring is usually carried out indiscriminately—many companies use "spyware" that throws up a red flag if someone on their network visits a pornographic or illegal Web site—but your boss can also have IT monitor you directly if he or she is so inclined. Either way, there's nothing you can do about it. The federal Electronic Communications Privacy Act gives your company the right to monitor all Internet, e-mail, and instant-messaging activity that occurs on your computer, regardless of whether you're sitting at your desk or connecting remotely to your office network from home. (If you're not connected to the office network, however, the company has no way to monitor you.)

Bottom line: Stick to gabbing in the break room and reading the newspaper, but watch out for video surveillance; 16 percent of companies use cameras to track on-the-job performance.

### I noticed a client sneezing. A few minutes later, my boss introduced her to me. Did I really have to shake her hand?

Suck it up and shake hands. If you don't, the prospect will wonder what's

**PERCENTAGE OF PEOPLE WHO HAVE HAD AN OFFICE ROMANCE: 58**

wrong with you, and your boss will be embarrassed. You can excuse yourself later to wash up.

**Our office morale is at an all-time low. How can I keep from getting sucked into the bitterness spiral?**

Swim like hell against the current. "The vast majority of folks suffer and endure. That's not a good thing," says Peter Wylie, PhD, an industrial psychologist in Washington, DC. "You have a huge amount of leverage over your own destiny. You may have to do something more painful than what you're going through now in order to change it, but you do have a choice." This doesn't necessarily mean you have to quit your job. Try these tips instead:

Assess and address the source of the morale destruction. "More often than not, it's one person at the root, [one] who has some power or responsibility but whose interpersonal skills suck," says Dr. Wylie.

If you've tried before to discuss your problem with this person, you're within your rights to go above him or her. "Sometimes just sitting down with a reasonable person who's in a position of power is all it takes," says Dr. Wylie, who notes that anger and frustration often come with not feeling in control—and while you may have no direct control over the situation, bringing it to the attention of those who do can make you feel better.

If there is no one with the ability to help you, then it's time to quit.

Until you reach that point, watch your mouth. "There's a difference between venting frustration, which we all need to do to varying degrees, and being a chronic complainer," says Dr. Wylie. "The latter doesn't lead to corrective action. It's not good problem solving; it's really unproductive and ineffective." If you've bitched for weeks without any plan for how to fix things, you're only making the situation worse—and probably getting on everyone's nerves.

**The new guy in the office just doesn't get it. Should I tell his boss? I don't want to look like I have a vendetta against him, but he's a tool around company clients.**

Office rule 1: Protect yourself. Office rule 1a: Protect the company. Office rule 2: Stay out of other people's business, unless it affects rule 1 or 1a.

### I quit my job, and they won't let me into my office. What things do I have a right to?

You should have taken what you needed before you quit. Generally, the company owns what you've produced for it and any information you have stored on its computer system. Files are tricky. The company can keep you from taking home business-contact information, but if you just want some family photos, you could ask them to burn a CD. Legally, you are entitled to your picture of Aunt Edna, that Snap-on calendar, and other precious desk mementos. If you must have them, offer to search your desk with a security guard present.

### I'm stuck working with this guy I really hate. How can I conquer my urge to strangle him?

Take it from me—and I've got more urges than a caged gorilla—cravings are too powerful to flat-out eliminate. Doesn't matter if they're physical, sexual, or maniacal. You have to find a slightly less satisfying, slightly more legal alternative. If he deserves it, strangle him, but do it by sending a lippy e-mail, by beating his tail on a project, or by toasting his transfer to another department over beers with fellow haters. Giving in to the urge a little, rather than trying to totally resist it, will help make it disappear.

### Where I work, vacations are treated like a sign of weakness. How can I slip away without being shamed by my workaholic bosses?

There are two ways to deflect the jealousy and the guilt trips as you leave for Bali. One, don't leave messes for someone else to clean up. And two, nobody will ever question the time you take away from the office as long as you consistently prove you've earned it while on the premises.

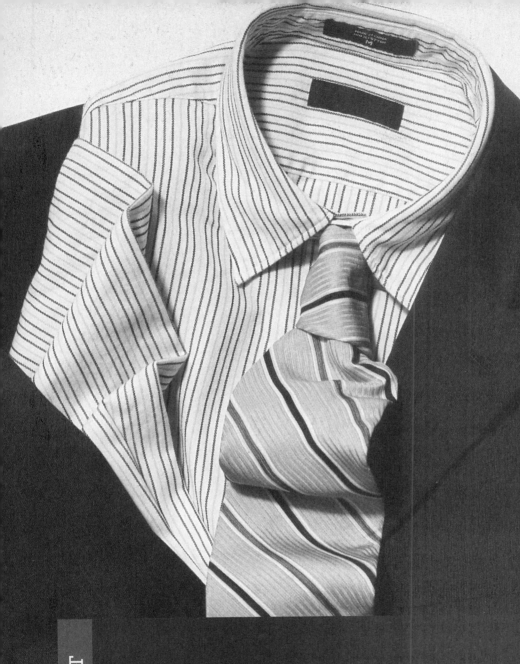

# EIGHT

# LOOK GREAT

# READ UP ON IT

## What Not to Wear

Six common style blunders and how to fix them

### by Clinton Kelly

A couple of years ago, I became cohost of TLC's *What Not to Wear*. Now it's a rare day that passes without at least one guy approaching me in public with the line "Hey, Clinton, I love your show!" followed by its now ridiculously predictable caveat, "My wife makes me watch it." I almost always smile and say, "Thank you," waiting for the inevitable next question: "So, what do you think of what I'm wearing?"

Invariably, I say, "You look great," and wish him well. But, more often than not, my gentlemen fans are guilty of fashion violations more galling than their propensity for barging in on a stranger's sushi dinner. (At least it won't get cold, right?) Here are just some of the things I'd tell them if I weren't so hell-bent on returning home with all my teeth.

**You are not an XXL.** I hate to break it to you, stud, but you're nowhere near as big as your clothes. Maybe you wouldn't look so much like Quasimodo if the shoulder seams on your shirt hit at—get this—your shoulders, rather than halfway down your arms. I have two words of counsel: large or (gulp) medium.

**Those pleats make you look like you have an estrogen imbalance.** A single pleat on each side of your pants can be perfectly acceptable, but any more and you're only adding volume to your crotch. And it's not the illusion of manly heft you're creating but more like a menopausal woman's "pooch."

**Your shoes suck.** They're scuffed and dirty and probably falling apart—which is too bad, because your suit looks halfway decent. Contrary to what you believe, everyone notices—and immediately makes a mental note that you do not take such great care of yourself. Do yourself (and your dogs) a favor: Buy some nice leather-soled lace-ups.

**I can see your balls.** Look, if you're competing in a triathlon, wear all the spandex you want. But let's be real: When you're doing your back-and-

**PERCENTAGE OF WOMEN WHO SAY THE FIRST THING THEY NOTICE ABOUT A MAN IS HIS HAIR:** 42

shoulders routine at the gym, chafing down there is not such a big issue. Nor is support. Throw a pair of shorts over those things.

**Your tie knot is dinky.** Some fashions require a small knot, as do men with smaller frames, for proportion's sake. But for most guys on most occasions, the knot you tied for your 13th birthday party—rabbit goes around the hole and back through—just doesn't cut it. Try a half Windsor. You can find instructions on the Internet, brainiac.

**Jerry Seinfeld has moved on.** White athletic sneakers and high-waisted jeans? Are you freakin' kidding me? Nobody does that anymore—except kids who were in diapers the first time around and now think it's cool to be retro. On you, it looks dated. Please realize that you are watching reruns—from a decade ago. It's time for an update.

# Corner-Office Bound

Eight sartorial strategies for putting your best foot forward

**edited by Matt Bean**

We asked 50 of the nation's top business leaders for their straight talk on style. Here's what these captains of industry said.

## HOW SHOULD I EXPRESS MYSELF IN AN OFFICE SETTING?

The CEOs say...

58% patterned neckwear and shirts
15% jewelry (rings, earrings, bracelets)
15% cuff links
5% whimsical neckwear

"Having great style is something people notice over the course of time. But having bad style is noticed immediately."
**Brett Fahlgren, director of special events, Prada**

**Match colors, mix patterns.** Your shirt and tie should share a shade. But if you're going to match patterns, "make sure they're a different scale," says Lynne Marks, president of Atlanta's London Image Institute. "For example, choose a larger pattern for your tie while keeping the shirt reserved."

**Avoid pattern blindness.** Your shirt and tie are the palette from which you paint the colors of your soul. Just keep the palette small. "A large pattern is far more casual than a small one, so if you work in a conservative office, stick to small checks and pinstripes," says Marks.

**Go light on the bling.** Just because you're the king of accounting doesn't mean you need to wear a diamond-studded tie clip. In addition to a dress watch and a stylish belt, "a nice signet ring or wedding ring is all you should wear," says Marks.

## WHAT'S THE MOST IMPORTANT ACCESSORY FOR A NEW HIRE?

The CEOs say...

50% well-polished shoes
18% a smart attaché case
15% an elegant watch
8% matching belt and shoes

"Who wants a sloppy employee in an era when you can go to jail for reporting incorrect financial data?"
**Tom Markert, global chief of marketing, ACNielsen**

**Shine with spit.** "It's that old military concept: Spit, polish, and repeat," says New York City shoemaker Warren Edwards. "You want to rub the polish in a circular motion—don't just slap it all over the shoe—then add some water and really polish hard."

**Cut the cream.** Wax-based polishes last longer. "Any wax will work better than the sponge-on liquid polish that everyone is selling these days," says Edwards. Select a brush with long, sturdy bristles.

**Store with care.** "Shoes will develop creases and the toes will turn up if you don't store them on trees," says Edwards. "Shoes are made on the principle of stretching leather. If you don't guide them back into place after they've been wet or you've worn them all day, they'll deform."

## WHAT SHOULD I WEAR TO DINNER WITH A CLIENT?

The CEOs say...

35% trousers, a dress shirt, and a sport coat
28% a suit and tie
28% jeans, a sport coat, and a dress shirt
8% a leather jacket, trousers, and a dress shirt

"Everybody wonders at some point whether they're going to be overdressed or underdressed. It's not some taboo discussion. Just ask."
**Mike Fasulo, chief marketing officer, Sony Electronics**

**Lighten up.** Unless you live in New York City or Berlin, wear blue or gray sport coats instead of black, says Michelle Sterling, of Global Image Group, an image consulting firm. "Black is too formal for business and can put people off," she says.

**Frame your face.** If you're opting for the open-collar look, be careful about your choice of shirt. Wide or round faces look best with long, pointed collars, and narrow faces require wider, spread collars. In between? Go either way.

**Pick the right kicks.** Basic loafers won't cut it with a suit or dressy trou-

**PERCENTAGE OF WOMEN WHO SAY A UNIBROW IS A TURNOFF: 84**

sers; wingtips and cap-toe shoes can be too dressy for khakis and cords. Your utility infielder: leather lace-ups. Look for a classic oxford style, says Guillermo Molina, an elite Manhattan tailor.

## HOW SHOULD I DRESS FOR A CREATIVE WORKPLACE?
The CEOs say...

36% trousers, a shirt, and a sweater
23% a suit, dress shirt, and tie
23% jeans, a shirt, and a sport coat
5% casual pants and a T-shirt

"It doesn't matter if you're working at a law firm or a rock club. Your image should be in step with the firm's attitudes and beliefs. Your clothes are part of your résumé."
**Steve Tetrault, president, Tetrault Design Associates**

**Don't dress down.** Just because you can get away with a T-shirt and flip-flops doesn't mean you should. The more casual the dress code, the greater the opportunity to showcase smart clothing choices. One option: Add a navy or black soft-shouldered sport jacket to a pair of jeans and a white dress shirt.

**Play it straight.** Business casual doesn't mean you can lose your dry cleaner's number. "Even wrinkle-free clothes look bad if you don't take them out of the dryer fast enough," says Pat Newquist, president of Wardrobe Image.com. Bonus tip: Install a hook in your office to hang your discarded layers on during the day.

**Hide your pits.** If your company allows you to wear a golf or polo shirt, look for one with banded sleeves. This extra detail looks cleaner and more finished, and it prevents your co-workers from ogling your pit hair, should you raise your arms above your chest.

## WHAT SHOULD I WEAR TO AN AWARDS EVENT?
The CEOs say...

75% a suit, dress shirt, and tie
10% trousers, a button-down shirt, and a sport coat
8% a suit and dress shirt
5% a tuxedo

"Attitude is important. Some people can't be convincing in French cuffs and a Gucci suit. You have to be able to pull off what you're wearing."
**Tim Story, director of *Fantastic Four***

**Stay fresh.** If it's an annual event, spring for a crisp, new white dress shirt. "They get dingy and yellow when you wear them on a regular basis," says Elena Castaneda, president of New York Image Consulting. To add a little color, go for light blue. Skip black unless you're Marilyn Manson or a Johnny Cash wannabe.

**Lose some buttons.** The more buttons, the dressier the suit—and the stuffier the look. One- and two-button suits are formal yet fashionable. If you do choose a three-button suit (the upper limit), never close the bottom button; whether you button just the top, just the middle, or both the top and middle buttons is up to you.

**Tie it right.** Wear a silver- or champagne-colored satin tie for formal events," says Sterling. Use a fat knot, such as a Windsor. For wild ties, make sure the pattern size matches your body scale. "If you have medium-size features, wear medium-size patterns, and so on," she says.

## WHAT'S THE MOST ACCEPTABLE LOOK FOR CASUAL FRIDAYS?

The CEOs say...

46% jeans and a button-down shirt
24% khakis, a polo shirt, and a sweater
10% a suit jacket, a collared shirt, and jeans
10% trousers, a collared shirt, and a sport coat

"If you look like you're ready to paint a house or repair a leaky roof, chances are you're a little too relaxed for the workplace."
**David Beigie, vice president of corporate communications, T-Mobile USA**

**Choose the right jeans.** Dark washes are more formal than lighter washes. The distressed look—holes, frayed edges, questionable discolorations around the groin—screams rock star, not rising star. Jeans should be pressed and smooth, even if it's just with a hand steamer.

PERCENTAGE OF WOMEN WHO THINK MEN SHOULDN'T SPEND MORE TIME GROOMING THAN WOMEN DO: **95**

**Throw in a formal touch.** "A pressed, long-sleeved shirt will add a layer of respect," says Rachel Dee, a Denver-based image consultant. Leave your clubbing shirt at home and keep your chest hair and any neck chains on lockdown—a couple of unfastened buttons should suffice.

**Watch your waistline.** A braided leather belt is like a time machine back to 1991, and a belt-clipped BlackBerry is the modern equivalent of the pocket protector. Choose a thin, solid-colored belt—nothing faded or distressed—to match your shoes. And holster the communicator elsewhere.

## WHAT SHOULD I WEAR TO PROJECT CONFIDENCE?

The CEOs say...

70% a well-tailored suit
18% a conservative shirt-and-tie combination
8% a power tie

"A new suit is like any other opportunity. The right tailoring shows you know how to follow through."
**Congressman Charlie Dent (Republican–PA)**

**Sculpt your shoulders.** "They're the first thing you see when you meet someone," says Molina. "If it's an old suit, ask the tailor to reconstruct the shoulders using felt shoulder caps. They're less severely shaped than those made of other fabrics. And if it's a new suit, buy for the shoulders, not the waistline or hips. Shoulders are harder to fix."

**Ditch the pleats.** One crease is enough. "The younger entrepreneurs, the guys who want to look sharp, they want flat-front pants," says Molina. "If a suit is too expensive to replace or has sentimental value, a good tailor can reconstruct the pants for about $100 to $150."

**Do a dry run.** When you're being fitted, wear the same shirt, undergarments, and shoes you'll wear with the finished suit. "It's common sense, but guys come in wearing T-shirts and sneakers all the time," says Molina.

## WHAT'S THE RIGHT OUTFIT FOR A COMPANY RETREAT?

The CEOs say...

36% khakis and a sport coat
23% trousers and a dress shirt
23% jeans and a sport shirt
3% shorts and a button-down shirt

"There's nothing like being stuck in the middle of nowhere with the wrong clothes for 3 days. Dressing for a corporate getaway is the hardest thing you can do."

**Lauren Solomon, former vice president of professional image development, Chase Manhattan Bank**

**Wear layers.** When in doubt, overdress. "You can always remove your sport coat," says Dee. Underneath it, you can even layer a sport shirt over a high-quality T-shirt that's the same color as a stripe in either your coat or your sport shirt.

**Choose the right khakis.** They're a casual middle ground between jeans and slacks, but one pair of khakis doesn't fit all. Lighter skin tones require lighter khakis, while darker complexions look best with darker khakis, says San Francisco Bay-area image consultant Anthea Tolomei.

**Watch the CEO for cues.** At dinner, watch the highest-ranking person in the room. If he or she shows up in a suit, you've come prepared. If the honcho shows up in jeans and a barn jacket, throw the sport coat over the back of your chair and roll up your sleeves.

# Closet Smarts

What to wear if you want your clothes torn off

**by Kathryn Eisman**

Boxers or briefs? Wingtips or loafers? Cashmere or leather? Inquiring minds wanted to know, so we asked some self-proclaimed experts—800 women— what they think you should wear…

## …TO BED

The ladies said:

42% boxers
34% nothing; sleep naked
11% boxers and T-shirt
9% pajama pants
3% pajama pants and T-shirt
Less than 1% flannel pajama set

Save your pj bottoms for solo nights. Women want sleeping companions in boxers, or nude. However, 58 percent of us prefer a man in boxer briefs for everyday wear. Go with cotton or microfiber, the sexiest-ranking fabrics, according to the ladies.

## …ON A FIRST DATE

The ladies said:

56% something casual but chic
27% casual Friday style (khakis or dress pants, dress shirt)
7% casual (jeans, T-shirt, hoodie)
6% straight from work (suit or blazer, minus the tie)
3% dressed to impress (suit, tie)

Show that you put some effort into what you're wearing (it says the date is important to you) but you're not trying too hard (which says you're desperate

**PERCENTAGE OF WOMEN WHO THINK CLEAN-SHAVEN MEN ARE SEXIEST: 58**

or, worse, slick). Slip on jeans and a cool, crisp shirt, and add a structured blazer. Oh, and make the blazer a soft fabric like corduroy, suede, or velvet; it gives her an excuse to touch you.

## ...TO MEET HER PARENTS
The ladies said:

48% casual Friday best
25% casual chic (jeans, dress shirt, blazer)
14% straight from work (suit or blazer, minus the tie)
9% dressed to impress (suit, tie)
4% casual (jeans, T-shirt, hoodie)

The goal: Look approachable and responsible. Wear conservative, neutral trousers with a soft-pastel shirt—maybe pink. (Forty-eight percent of women say a man in a pink shirt is "hot and confident.") Add a sport coat and you'll look honorable, even if your intentions are anything but.

## ...ON YOUR FEET
The ladies said:

26% leather loafers
15% dress boots
14% trainers
14% wingtip dress shoes
13% running shoes
9% leather sandals
8% rubber flip-flops
7% cowboy boots

Women size up a man's shoes as indicators of his overall sense of style, social status, and cash flow. What we see in the man in loafers is a casual elegance that hints at a sensual life of sauvignon blanc on the beach and lazy Sunday breakfasts in bed.

## ...ON YOUR BUTT
The ladies said:

54% faded vintage-style jeans
34% dark, clean denim
5% tight, George Michael style

4% baggy, hip-hop style

3% ripped, rock 'n' roll style

With proper care, a pair of jeans, like a relationship, can last a lifetime. Maybe that explains why we love seeing your butt covered in worn-in denim, a spot of thigh showing through a hole. You seem like you'd be a loyal boyfriend who won't throw us away at the first sign of fraying. Top with a bright sweater, the perfect contrast to your blues.

## ...FOR FABRIC

The ladies said:

33% cashmere

27% leather

11% wool

10% suede

10% silk

7% corduroy

2% velvet

The contrast of a rough man in supersoft cashmere is irresistible. Also, 63 percent of women say a man in a scarf is hot, and 23 percent think green is a color you should wear more often.

# S C I - G U Y

## Get More Face Time

The more often a woman sees your face, the better it will look to her. The brain favors familiar faces when choosing a partner, according to a new study from the University of Liverpool in the United Kingdom. Researchers showed more than 200 men and women photos of faces that had been digitally altered to move the eyes closer together or farther apart. When asked later to compare the attractiveness of two faces, those who had viewed the wide-eyed visages tended to choose the wide-eyed image; those who'd viewed the faces with close-set eyes preferred a similar look. Study author Anthony Little, PhD, says the research reveals that "the brain has some flexibility in deciding what is and what isn't attractive." Little's previous research illustrated that a man is more likely to choose a partner with hair and eye color similar to his mother's.

## Go Deep

Don't expect a soul-melding moment at first blush. A study of speed daters found that men and women determine interest in dating partners based almost solely on physical appearance. University of Pennsylvania researchers reviewed data from 10,526 people participating in HurryDate, a service in which people decide in 3 minutes whether they want to go out with each other. Shocker: Women like tall, handsome types; men tend to judge based on weight. "Women act just like men in these situations; they go pretty much entirely by looks," says Jason Weeden, PhD. So find a scene that allows the real you to shine, he says: work, cultural or charity events, athletics.

## Fight Fat and Win

Think you're so charming that women won't mind your gut? Fat chance. A new University of Washington study says excessive weight is more of a turnoff than an STD is when it comes to choosing a mate. More than 400 male and female college students ranked drawings of potential sex partners. Women found men who were infected with an STD more appealing than men who were obese. Men were even harsher about weight, rating overweight women lower than those who were afflicted with an STD or a physical disability. "In a country where 65 percent of people are overweight, having thinness as an important criterion is problematic," says study author Eunice Chen, PhD. "Men are really narrowing their chances of having a relationship."

## Parlez-Vous?

A recent survey shows that speaking a foreign language makes you more attractive. Now consider this: A Japanese panel of experts in psychology and sociology developed the ultimate romantic line: "*Rainen no kono hi mo issho ni waratteiyoh.*" Translation: "This time next year, let's be laughing together." John Nathan, PhD, a professor of Japanese cultural studies at the University of California at Santa Barbara, says the line could work in Japan but warns, "American women might be a little less gullible."

## Find Common Ground

Little things do mean a lot. Trivial things like shared birthdays, having the same first initial, or having similar-sounding names make people more attractive, researchers report in the *Journal of Personality and Social Psychology*. Charles pairs with Charlotte, Pete with Paula. You see someone else born March 22 as The One because that's your birthday. The scientific explanation is "implicit egotism." Translation: We like ourselves, so we also tend to subconsciously like whatever reminds us of ourselves (people, places, and things)—no matter how minor the "connection."

## Pump Up Your Ego

Don't let the mirror be your measure of a workout's effectiveness. Research in the journal *Body Image* shows that women and men differ in the way they perceive themselves. In the study of 44 men and women, ages 18 to 29, researchers assessed the participants' body image, fat, muscularity, and

AMOUNT MEN SPENT ON GROOMING PRODUCTS IN 2005: **$4 billion** strength at the beginning and end of a 12-week resistance-training program. The women scored higher on body-image assessments after seeing an increase in the amount of weight they could lift. Men's body image improved only when they thought they looked better. Study author Kathleen Martin Ginis, PhD, recommends tracking how much weight you're lifting or how far you're running, so you can focus more on your body's achievements and less on your jeans size.

## Keep Your Teeth

If finding time to get outdoors is like pulling teeth, at least you'll know what to expect down the road. According to a new report from the Washington University School of Medicine, a vitamin D deficiency due to insufficient sun exposure could hasten your need for dentures. That's because the shortfall leads to bone loss as well as increased inflammation, a symptom of periodontal diseases, says Charles Hildebolt, PhD, the study author. Spending just 15 minutes in direct sunlight twice a week can provide you—and your teeth—with all the vitamin D you need. Or you can effortlessly supplement by drinking fortified milk and brushing with a fortified toothpaste, such as Sea Fresh.

## Brush with Greatness

Want the best brush for your buck? Power toothbrushes remove plaque and reduce the risk of gum disease better than ordinary manual ones. When researchers from the University of Sheffield in the United Kingdom reviewed 42 oral-health studies of nearly 4,000 people, they found that those who used oscillating power brushes had 11 percent less plaque and 6 percent less gum inflammation over 1 to 3 months than those who used manual brushes. After 3 months they had 17 percent less gingivitis, too. "You do not need to buy a powered toothbrush to clean your teeth well," says Peter Robinson, PhD, the study author, "but if you want the best performance, a powered brush with a rotation oscillation action is the best to buy." Try one of those used in the study: Braun Oral-B ProfessionalCare 7000 series. (about $60, www.oralb.com)

## Fight Wrinkles with Food

Spending a buck or two at the vitamin store may banish all of those fine lines and wrinkles you've been trying to ignore. According to a study published in

*Free Radical Biology and Medicine,* beta-carotene—an antioxidant found in carrots, fruits, and green leafy vegetables like spinach—helps counter fine lines and wrinkles. In tests with human skin cells, beta-carotene suppressed the proteins that digest skin collagen and cause premature aging from ultraviolet radiation. "You could call beta-carotene a very gentle internal sun protector," says study author Regina Goralczyk, who recommends consuming 4 to 6 milligrams a day. One easy way to get it: Pop a supplement. Look for one that contains at least 4 milligrams, and be sure to take it with food. Beta-carotene is a fat-soluble vitamin; without fat to help your body digest it, there's no benefit.

## Change Your Meds

Clear skin could lead to a clogged nose. Taking antibiotics for acne doubles a person's risk of catching a cold, says a study in the *Archives of Dermatology.* After monitoring more than 118,000 pimple-prone adults for 15 years, researchers found that the people on oral antibiotics were twice as likely to develop upper-respiratory infections as were those given other treatments. The reason? Antibiotics can annihilate the body's "good" bacteria, which help fight invading viruses. Even topical antibiotics can kill protective bacteria in the nose, mouth, and throat, says lead author David Margolis, MD, PhD. If you have acne, ask your dermatologist for prescription benzoyl peroxide or Retin-A (tretinoin) cream instead.

# WHAT'S NEW

## Longer Life Jacket

A high-tech jacket protects you from the harshest climates on the planet, but it may not survive your washing machine's spin cycle. Clean your jacket incorrectly and the breathable, waterproof fabric will sop up fluids like a frat boy at his first kegger. Don't just throw your jacket in the wash with your sweat socks. Typical laundry detergents interfere with waterproofing. Instead, use Granger's 2 in 1 cleaning and waterproofing product (www.grangersusa.com). If water doesn't bead on the garment's surface, "it's time for a waterproofing treatment," says Dennis Lewon, *Backpacker®* magazine's gear guru. "Usually, you have to treat a jacket about once a year."

## Hot Steam Machine

Washing machines hog water and power, two things we can't afford to waste. The LG Tromm SteamWasher cuts down on both; it also zaps germs with a midwash blast of hot steam. It won't waste your time, either: Throw in your clothes—even if they're dry-clean only—for a quick steam cycle, and you'll rid them of odors and creases without subjecting them to a full wash. (about $1,500, www.lgusa.com)

## Gillette Fusion Razor

Time for our annual razor recap: First came Gillette's triple-blade Mach3, and it was great. Then Schick responded with the four-blade Quattro, and it was better. Then Gillette added a AA battery to the Mach3, and it vibrated, razing facial hair like redwoods and leaving barren skin behind. We loved it! This year, Gillette added—ready for this?—two more blades. And, we must admit, there's nothing like sweeping a phalanx of five blades across your mug. You're an alpha male; this is an alpha razor. Plus, a trimmer blade on the back of the razor cartridge makes delicate facial maneuvers a cinch. (about $10, www.gillette.com)

# Tooth Whitener

Many tooth-whitening products can make your teeth sensitive to heat and cold, but a new type of whitener reduces sensitivity, according to American Dental Association (ADA) scientists. Bleaching typically widens tiny pores in your enamel, making the teeth sensitive, but the new product replaces minerals that teeth naturally lose, which decreases sensitivity, says Frederick Eichmiller, DDS, director of the ADA's Paffenbarger Research Center. A *Journal of the American Dental Association* study reports that people who used whiteners and a gel containing calcium and phosphate to replace lost minerals were twice as likely as the placebo group to be pain-free. These whiteners with added minerals are available at most dental practices, and they're worth asking about if you've tried bleaching in the past and had problems with sensitivity, Dr. Eichmiller says. His team is working on combining the two key ingredients into a gel or strip to be sold over the counter. It could be out of the lab in a year.

# T A K E 5

## Mix and Match

Five keys to mixing patterns and colors

Never mix patterns. That's the conventional wisdom you've been hearing for years. And it's fine if you want to look, well, conventional. But if you want to stand out and show some personality, you need to learn how to smartly pair interesting patterns and hues. It's easier than it looks. "Part of it is on-the-spot creativity," says Brian Boyé, *Men's Health* fashion director. "With great style, some rules are meant to be broken. Still, there are a few easy guidelines."

**Invest in key pieces.** "A pin-striped suit is a great starting point, because it gives you a background," says Michael Macko, men's fashion director for Saks Fifth Avenue. "Then you can have fun with shirts, ties, and pocket squares, because there are a ton out there in different patterns and price ranges." Add the following to your closet for optimal mixing possibilities:

1. Windowpane dress shirt
2. Striped sweater
3. Polka-dotted pocket square
4. Repp striped tie
5. Paisley tie
6. Argyle sweater
7. Pin-striped suit
8. Chalk-striped suit
9. Windowpane sport coat
10. Striped socks

**Stay neutral.** "The more subtle the color palette, the easier it is to get away with mixing different patterns," says Macko. "I always try to ground everything in a neutral—maybe a navy, gray, or tan." If you work in a creative workplace, give brighter colors a try. If a mixed-pattern look is too busy for your office, express yourself more subtly with your tie selection. "You can wear a solid gray suit with a pale blue or pink shirt, but then your tie is something you can really have fun with," says Macko.

**Recruit a critic.** When in doubt, don't wear a combination. "Sometimes mixing patterns is a bit of a risk, and the worst thing is to feel self-conscious about what you're wearing," says Macko. If possible, ask a partner or roommate for a second opinion.

**Show your stripes.** If your jacket has fine pinstripes, wear a tie or shirt with bold, thick stripes. When the different stripes are too close in size, a viewer's eye doesn't know where to focus. Mixing is all about scale.

**Check yourself.** The same rule applies with checks—make sure one is significantly larger than the other. That said, a windowpane dress shirt with a small-checked tie always looks better than vice versa.

# MEN'S HEALTH
# Q       U       I       Z

## Are You a Style Guru?

Take our test to see if you know a thing or two about clothes but ignore the most important consideration of all: self-knowledge

### 1. Do your clothes complement your coloring?
A. Your skin and hair tones are very similar.
B. The difference between your hair and skin colors is a little more pronounced.
C. Your hair is dark and your skin is light.

If your skin and hair tones are very similar (A), you have a muted complexion. Choose tops in a soft, monotone color format to complement your coloring, advises Alan Flusser, owner of Alan Flusser Custom Shop in New York City and author of *Dressing the Man*. Wearing high-contrast coloring, such as black and white, near your face will dilute your natural pigmentation and distract the viewer's eye. For suits, choose midnight navy instead of black. A dress shirt in a medium shade of blue will bring out blue eyes more effectively than a pale blue shirt.

If the difference between your hair and skin colors is a little more pronounced (B), you have a medium-contrast complexion. Medium-contrast men can experiment with almost any medium-to-strong color combination to strengthen their complexions.

If your hair is dark and your skin is light (C), you have a high-contrast complexion. Surround your face with contrasting colors of equal strength to enliven your face's natural vitality, says Flusser. You can wear black and white together to good effect.

Note that the complexion of African-American men is not considered muted because when a white shirt surrounds a dark face (regardless of shade), considerable contrast results. If you have dark skin, follow the advice for medium- or high-contrast complexions. Tyson Beckford has a very high-contrast complexion—so the brighter and more dramatic the shade of his clothes, the better he looks and the more striking his skin tone.

# DON'T BE A DON'T

Here are three fashion faux pas, according to Brian Boyé, *Men's Health* fashion director.

**Don't look like a clown.** Mixing three patterned items at one time (such as a shirt, tie, and jacket) is the limit.

**Don't overaccessorize.** When you combine patterns and colors, your clothes make a bold style statement, so keep accessories like your belt and shoes simple and the same color.

**Don't forget your proportions.** Big guys: Keep in mind that large patterns will enhance your bigness. Small guys: Bold patterns can add desired bulk to your frame.

**2. Is your shirt making the right point?**
A. Your face is round like a basketball or wide like a football.
B. Your face is narrow.
C. You have a long neck.

There are an infinite number of shirt-collar combinations, each for a different body type. Choose a collar based on the shape of your face and the length of your neck.

If your face is round like a basketball or wide like a football (A), choose a straight-point collar 3 inches long, which will lengthen your appearance. Stay away from spread collars, which will only accentuate the width. For the best examples of this style, look for shirts by Perry Ellis, Giorgio Armani, Claiborne, and Hathaway. With a narrow collar, keep your tie knot small.

If your face is narrow (B), a spread collar with a half-Windsor tie knot will balance it. Try Tommy Hilfiger, Robert Talbott, and Banana Republic. Spread-collar shirts are increasingly the shirt of choice for businessmen and are best when worn with a tie. Woven, as opposed to printed, ties make thicker, chunkier knots.

If your neck is long (C), wear a high collar, such as one from Dolce & Gabbana. These shirts stand up well under a jacket when worn without a tie; they won't creep down below your lapel as the day or evening wears on.

**3. Are your shoes sending the same signal as your clothes?** It's casual Friday, and you're wearing khakis and a button-down. You plan to wear . . .

    A. Black wingtips
    B. Brown loafers
    C. Casual boots

Answer: B or C. Wingtips are meant for suits only. Casual pants call for casual shoes.

### 4. Should you wear cuffed pants?
    A. Are you under 5 foot 10?
    B. Are the pants khakis, cords, or microfiber trousers?
    C. Are you dressing for a casual evening out?
    D. Do you wear flat-front pants?

Answer: Don't wear cuffs if you answered yes to any of the above. The only exception is if you wear business formal clothing to the office. Cuffed trousers are a polished look that will serve you well in the boardroom. "Sophisticated men wear cuffs on their pants, and other sophisticated men notice," says Andy Gilchrist, author of *Andy's Encyclopedia of Men's Clothes*. "Cuffs are de rigueur with pleated pants, especially suit trousers."

# BURNING QUESTIONS

### What about a man says "classy" to a woman?

A gentleman is a class act, and a class act knows how to make others feel comfortable, says *How to Be a Gentleman* author John Bridges. Hold doors open, pull out chairs, and offer your coat when it's cold. But any obvious flourishes will flush you out as a fake. Pay attention to the subtle, because she'll notice things like...

**Your nails.** You don't need a manicure, but there's nothing feminine about cleaning your nails and clipping them to subfeline length, says Bridges.

**Your eating skills.** For cutting, the fork is held in your left hand, and the knife is held in your right hand. Once your knife has been used, it should not touch the linen; lay it across your dinner plate if you need to set it down.

**Your neighborhood cred.** Foster relationships with neighborhood establishments, like the local pub, indie bookstore, and corner deli, long before the date, say Phineas Mollod and Jason Tesauro, authors of *The Modern Gentleman: A Guide to Essential Manners, Savvy & Vice*. Taking a date to places where everyone knows your name lends credibility to the notion that you're not feigning the nice-guy act to get in her pants. It also shows you have roots in your community, and when it comes to roots—as with biceps—the stronger, the better.

### Are black jeans just as acceptable as blue? If so, what can I wear with them?

Yes, you can wear black jeans anywhere you'd sport blue denim. While black jeans may appear dressier than their casual blue counterparts, they're still jeans and therefore are not a stand-in for your smart black trousers. And, unlike blue jeans, which get better with age, black jeans should remain solid black. Once yours start fading into acid-wash, it's time to throw them out.

### I have a rather large backside. What's the best way to cover it up?

Lower-rise pants with boot-cut ankles will shorten the apparent length and breadth of your buttocks. Skip the beige slacks—dark colors are more forgiving—and avoid pleats. If you tuck shirts into your trousers, keep the shirts on the shorter side for less bulk beneath the belt. If all else fails, cover up with a ventless jacket.

### What do women think of a city guy in cowboy boots?

They're afraid he wants to hog-tie them.

### Will I look stupid in motorcycle-inspired clothing if I've never ridden a bike?

Probably. The trick is to look motorcycle inspired, not obsessed. Keep it to one biker item per outfit. A jacket, for instance. Look for something with the standard style accents—the shorter-than-usual length, zip-up front, rugged leather, and tough hardware detailing—but ditch the padded shoulders and belted waist. Pair it with denim jeans and a cotton T-shirt.

### What's a good look for a barbecue at a friend's house? Everyone wears printed shirts with flames running up the sides.

Suede slides or nice Italian loafers are your foundation. Next: white jeans. Add a clean-cut gingham shirt for the preppy look, a vintage-inspired printed tee for the hipster look, or a slim-fitting floral shirt to go Euro.

### What's the deal with printed socks? Lame? Are there any rules?

Save the printed socks for the rich, eccentric Englishman who hunts foxes, smokes a pipe, and says "exquisite" far too frequently. Stick to solids and subdued patterns.

### Wide-flared and boot-cut jeans are everywhere. What's the best look?

Flared pants are best left hanging in the Rock and Roll Hall of Fame. But the subtler boot-cut jeans can work wonders for the average man. The wider cut at the ankle can balance out thicker thighs and add a little panache to your typical weekend wear. The flare should be barely noticeable. If you start looking like an extra in *Saturday Night Fever,* I can guarantee you'll be spending your Saturday nights at home.

**PERCENTAGE OF WOMEN WHO WEAR THEIR HUSBAND'S CLOTHES: 56**

## PERCENTAGE OF HUSBANDS WHO WEAR THEIR WIFE'S CLOTHES: 16

### What's the right length for a T-shirt?

Some men wear T-shirts that are so long they could be mistaken for dresses. Worse is a short tee—no one needs to see your happy trail. The perfect T-shirt falls just below your hips, or a couple of inches below the top of your pants. To test, lift your arms over your head. No belly showing? You're in business.

### My tailor asked me whether I wanted cuffs on a suit I was having altered. Are there any rules?

Cuffs add weight to the bottom of the trousers, allowing your pants legs to drape better and flow when you walk. As a general rule, if the pants have pleats, they need cuffs. If they're flat-front, skip the cuffs and opt for a hem instead.

# INDEX

Boldface page references indicate photographs. Underscored references indicate boxed text.

## A

Abdominal fat, 15, 25
Abs
  body-fat percentage and, 27
  of Brad Pitt, 52
  building, 21, 23–24, 52
  quiz on, 23–26
A-B Split workout, 75
Abstention from sex, 86, 99
ACE inhibitors, 192
Aceon (perindopril erbumine), 192
Acid reflux, 142, 250
Acne, 121–22, 282
Acomplia (rimonabant), 19
Acupuncture, 128, 167
Adenosine, 191
Aerobic capacity, 63
Age
  childbearing and, 229
  muscle loss and, 33
  sex and, 106
  tips on staying young and, 38
Age-related macular degeneration, 128
Agility, 54–55, 54
Air pollution, 217
Alarm clock for tracking sleep patterns, 132
Alcohol
  abdominal fat and, 25
  in Alzheimer's disease prevention, 200
  atrial fibrillation and, 169
  cholesterol and, 18, 193
  muscles and, 77
  prostate cancer prevention and, 189
  testosterone and, 25, 77
  weight loss and, 18
Aller-7, 131
Allergies, 131
Allicin, 194
Alzheimer's disease
  dementia and, 180
  education and, 201
  hypertension drugs and, 192
  preventing
    alcohol, 200
    diet, 201
    exercise, 199–200
    prescription drugs, 192
  quiz on, 199–201
  senses and, 200
  Tylenol and, 199
  work and, 200
Ambien, 126
Androgen deprivation, 159
Androstenes, 95
Anesthetics, 137
Angiogram, 166, 168, 170–71
Ankle-brachial index, 204
Anthocyanins, 167, 191
Antibiotics
  arrhythmia and, 191
  bronchitis and, 128
  colds and, 282
  for sore throat, 120
Antidepressants, 13–14, 197
Antifungal creams, 121, 135
Antigen test, 120
Antioxidants, 189, 199, 282
Appearance and attraction. *See also* Clothing; Dental care; Grooming
  body fat, 279–80
  body image, 280–81
  eating skills, 291
  face, 279
  foreign language, speaking, 280
  hair, 136–37, 268
  new trends in, 283–84
  overweight, 279–80
  physical, 279
  questions about, 291–93
  relationships with neighborhood establishments, 291
  trivial things, 280
Appetite-suppression pill, 19
Aqua Touch Vibe, 84
Arrhythmia, 163, 191. *See also* Atrial fibrillation

prescription drugs for fighting, 194
skin, 121–22
testicular, 194, 206
Cannabinoid receptors, 19
Capoten (captopril), 192
Capsaicin, 167
Captopril (Capoten), 192
Car, when to buy new, 238
Car accidents, 197–98
Carbohydrates
    blood-sugar level and, 7
    breads and, 27
    fast-digesting, 7
    high-sugar, 8
    insulin and, 37
    intake of, average daily, 5
    slow-digesting, 8–9
    after workouts, 10, 38
Carboplatin, 194
Career. See Work
Carotid arteries, 203–4
Carotid ultrasound test, 203
Cartilage loss, 120
Cash flow, 237
Castration, chemical, 153, 159
Catechins, 16
Cavities, filling tooth, 131–32
Cell phones
    blood-alcohol level detection and, 131
    for children, 232
    medication reminders and, 131
    randy rings for, 97
    sperm and, 212
Celsius diet beverage, 19
Cereals, 4, 14
C-fiber nerves, 133
Charmin Ultra or Aloe & E toilet paper, 135
Cheese, 143
Chef Jay's Tri-O-Plex meal-replacement bar,
        29
Chemotherapy, 158, 194
Children
    age of childbearing and, 229
    beverages for, 214
    cell phones for, 232
    cleaning bathroom and, 221
    depression and, 231–32
    diet and, 214–15
    doctor visits and, 219
    eating out and, 218
    food introductions to, 218
    parenting and
        being there for, 210, 221, 224
        connecting with, 230–31

cost of raising child to age 18 and, 217
    disciplining, 224, 226, 230
    fitness, 214–15
    lessons taught and, 227
    life's transitions, 225–26
    listening to, 223
    overweight, 231
    playing with, 218–19, 222, 226, 226
    quality time, 227
    remarriage and, 231
    teenagers, 223–24, 223
portion control and, 218
teenaged, 223–24, 223, 231–32
tree house for, building, 222
as weight-loss saboteurs, 13
Chocolate, 93, 115
Cholesterol
    alcohol and, 18, 193
    HDL, 18, 167, 172, 203
    heart disease and, 164–65, 171–72
    LDL, 122, 164, 167, 170, 171–72, 177, 193,
        203
    measuring, 203
    triglycerides and, 170, 190, 203
    visceral fat and, 177
Chromosomes, 218
Ciclopirox gel, 121
Cigarettes, 197, 205, 217, 230
Cilostazol, 122
Circadian rhythm, 24
Circulatory problems, 122
Cisapride (Propulsid), 191
CLA, 21, 127–28
Clarithromycin, 191
Clif Bar, 28
Climax. See Orgasms
Clitoral contact and stimulation, 82, 104
Clock diet, 7–10, 7
Clothing. See also Shoes
    for barbecue at friend's house, 292
    bedtime, 106, 275
    butts and, 276–77, 291–92
    cleaning, 283
    color of, 285–86, 287
    fabrics, 253, 277
    finances and, 241–42
    for first date, 275–76
    jackets, high-tech, 283
    jeans, 291–92
    key pieces, 285
    for meeting her parents, 276
    men who wear wife's, 293
    mistakes, 288
    mixing and matching, 285–86